Solution-Focused Brief Practice with Long-Term Clients in Mental Health Services
"I Am More Than My Label"

Solution-Focused Brief Practice with Long-Term Clients in Mental Health Services
"I Am More Than My Label"

Joel K. Simon, MSW
Thorana S. Nelson, PhD

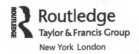

Routledge
Taylor & Francis Group
New York London

First published 2007 by The Haworth Press

Published 2021 by Routledge
605 Third Avenue, New York, NY 10017
2 Park Square, Milton Park, Abingdon, Oxon OX14 4RN

Routledge is an imprint of the Taylor & Francis Group, an informa business

PUBLISHER'S NOTE
The development, preparation, and publication of this work has been undertaken with great care. However, the Publisher, employees, editors, and agents of The Haworth Press are not responsible for any errors contained herein or for consequences that may ensue from use of materials or information contained in this work The Haworth Press is committed to the dissemination of ideas and information according to the highest standards of intellectual freedom and the free exchange of ideas Statements made and opinions expressed in this publication do not necessarily reflect the views of the Publisher, Directors, management. or staff of The Haworth Press or an endorsement by them.

Cover design by Marylouise E. Doyle

Library of Congress Cataloging-in-Publication Data

Simon, Joel K
    Solution-focused brief practice with long-term clients in mental health services . I am more than my label / Joel K. Simon, Thorana S Nelson
        p. ; cm.
    Includes bibliographical references.
    ISBN· 978-0-7890-2794-8 (hard : alk paper)
    ISBN 978-0-7890-2795-5 (soft . alk. paper)
    1. Brief psychotherapy 2. Mental health services. I Nelson. Thorana Stiever II Title
    [DNLM: 1 Psychotherapy, Brief—methods. 2. Mental Health Services 3. Professional-Patient Relations. WM 420.5.P5 S595s 2007]

    RC480 55 S57 2007
    616.89'14—dc22

                                                                            2007015530

ISBN 13: 978-0-7890-2795-5 (pbk)

To my companion, friend, and wife of 36 years, Joanna.
JKS

For Vic, who supports me in all that I do.
TSN

ABOUT THE AUTHORS

Joel K. Simon, CSW-R, BCD, ACSW, is Director of Social Work and Support Services at the Hospice of Orange and Sullivan Counties in Newburgh, New York. With over 27 years of experience as a therapist, clinical supervisor, program manager, trainer, and consultant, Mr. Simon is the author of several solution-focused articles and a founding member and webmaster of the Solution-Focused Brief Therapy Association. He is a licensed New York State social worker, a board certified diplomate in clinical social work, and a member of the National Association of Social Workers and of the Academy of Certified Social Workers.

Thorana S. Nelson, PhD, is Professor of Marital and Family Therapy in the Department of Family, Consumer, and Human Development at Utah State University, Logan. Dr. Nelson has been practicing family therapy for over 24 years and is a clinical member and approved supervisor of AAMFT. She is a founding member and sits on the Board of Directors of the Solution-Focused Brief Therapy Association, and a member of the American Family Therapy Academy.

CONTENTS

Foreword

Many years ago I worked at an adult community-based residential treatment center that specialized in working with people who had been labeled as schizophrenic or manic depressive following one or more psychiatric hospitalizations. As I read *Solution-Focused Brief Practice with Long-Term Clients in Mental Health Services,* I found myself remembering one of the clients in that program, a young woman who was then in her early thirties.

I initially got to know Sheila while leading a group at the community-based residential treatment center where she then lived. When we first met, Sheila was polite, but did not speak much unless directly asked a question. She kept her eyes down and walked with her shoulders hunched inward. She exchanged small talk with the people around her, but for the most part was silent. She appeared to spend all of her free time watching television while munching on bags of potato chips.

After I got to know her better, Sheila confided that the medication had affected her metabolism, causing her to feel tired and hungry most of the time regardless of what she ate and how much she slept. She explained that although she had gained a great amount of weight in the past year and didn't like the way her body looked, she was not interested in going on a diet because food was one of the few things that comforted her now. The way she said this suggested that she once had many more comforts in her life than she had now.

As I got to know her better, I learned that Sheila was mourning two losses: the loss of the professional career she had begun and the demise of her marriage. Both had been casualties of the psychiatric problems that had surfaced just a little over a year after her college graduation. Despite that the history documented in her treatment file contained little more than a list of past and current medications, dates of hospitalization, and meager references to her diagnosis of manic depression, Sheila's larger history was poignantly rich. She had re-

Solution-Focused Brief Practice

ceived high marks in a variety of subjects at the university, and her past experiences included membership in a sorority; volunteer work through her church; foreign travel; playing volleyball, baseball, and field hockey on recreational teams; an active social life with her friends; and marrying the man she had thought of as her soul mate. Following graduation, she had gotten a good job. Sheila had relished getting up each morning and going to work every day until the day she realized that she was no longer able to concentrate well enough to do her job. She had been fired that same week.

People in the small town where Sheila lived seemed to avoid her in the weeks following her first psychiatric hospitalization. The medication she had been given when she left the hospital made her groggy and left her limbs feeling stiff and uncomfortable. She found it difficult to concentrate well enough to read the newspaper, much less the novels she had once loved. She was no longer a member of any sports teams, and her former gardening hobby no longer gave her pleasure. She began spending all of her time indoors, alone.

Sheila looked forward to her husband's return from work each night, but his arrival was almost always a disappointment. The closeness they had once shared was gone. He seemed distant and preoccupied, expressed little interest in her, and he was often late. They argued about household chores such as cooking, cleaning, and laundry. He bitterly resented the debts they had incurred as a result of her hospitalization. The once tidy house they shared was now cluttered and dirty, and Sheila remained in the bedroom when her in-laws dropped by, too embarrassed to face them with her house in such disorder. It was a struggle to bathe and dress each morning, and some days she simply stayed in bed. Everyday life began to feel more and more impossible, and the medication did not seem to be helping.

Just when Sheila was convinced that things couldn't get worse, her husband confessed that he had been having an affair with the woman Sheila had formerly thought of as her best friend. When her husband told her that their marriage was over, Sheila decided to return to her former hometown and live with her parents for a few months until she got back on her feet.

Moving back in with her parents as an adult proved more difficult than Sheila had initially anticipated. She missed her independence, her job, and her friends even more than before. She felt as if the past few years of her adult life had been more or less erased, as if they had never existed, and that now her only identity was that of "psychiatric patient." A few months later, she was back in the inpatient psychiatric unit of the hospital. Rather than returning to her parents' home again, Sheila had elected to live at the community-based residential treatment center.

Sheila told me that the previous two-year interval, in which she had progressively lost her job, marriage, and friends, returned to her parents' home, and suffered the humiliation of two psychiatric hospitalizations, were the worst two years of her life. She confided that she had a deep fear of having a relapse, and strongly emphasized that she would rather die than go through something such as this ever again.

When Sheila described the hell she had experienced, I asked how she managed to keep going. She answered that she had not yet given up hope that she would someday be able to live on her own again like a normal person and have a cat or maybe a dog, some friends, and a job. These became our treatment goals.

I eventually stopped working at the residential treatment center and Sheila asked if she could continue to see me individually. She had just moved into a group home. We met once or twice a month for the next year, occasionally more often during times when she felt stressed, such as holidays, problems at work, and following visits home. Eventually Sheila moved out of the group home, and succeeded in getting her own apartment. She risked losing her disability checks by acquiring a part-time job in a bakery, explaining that working gave her a sense of self-worth.

We continued to meet for our sessions once or twice a month. I had cats back then and Sheila would always pause and pet one of them for a few minutes following our sessions. She would sigh and talk longingly about how much she missed living somewhere where she was allowed to keep a pet.

Our sessions were becoming less and less frequent by then. We met every six weeks and then eventually every eight weeks, and then every twelve weeks, and we eventually terminated therapy, although she continued to see her psychiatrist every other month for brief medication checks. Our only contact in the ensuing six months was one brief phone conversation in which she asked my advice about whether to attend an art therapy class that appealed to her and I expressed my support.

I was therefore quite surprised when Shiela showed up in front of my house a few months later while I was outside mowing the front lawn. She gestured to me and I turned off the lawnmower in order to hear what she was saying. Sheila explained that she happened to be passing by because she had just signed a lease on an apartment in the neighborhood. She was excited because it was a place that would allow pets. I noticed then that she was carrying a cat in her arms, a frag-- ile, forlorn looking creature that looked like it had done some hard living before Sheila had rescued it. Sheila then explained that she had rented an apartment in the building directly behind my house.

I remember flinching inwardly when Sheila first told me this, and to this day I fervently hope that my first reaction was not visible to her. Even twenty years later, I still feel shame at the initial apprehension I felt back then at the idea that a "mentally ill person" was moving practically next door. Most of the apprehension dissolved a moment later when I noticed that Sheila's eyes were shining with hope as she stood there looking at me, lovingly stroking the cat. I found myself admiring her courage and determination and finally remembering my manners, said something such as, "Congratulations. Welcome to the neighborhood." Then I asked her what she had named the cat.

Of course, I now realize that I needn't have worried about Sheila living nearby, nor would anyone else need to worry about this. Not surprisingly Sheila proved to be a courteous and pleasant neighbor, and she was an exemplary pet owner, volunteering at the local Humane Society, and taking excellent care of Tabby (not the cat's real name), whose once cloudy eyes and scrappy coat became clear and shiny with obvious good health. In the years before I moved away, I occasionally ran into Sheila at art fairs, outdoor concerts, and other events, although rarely on the block outside my house and we would exchange a few words.

It was apparent that she had many friends and interests, and that she had found a way to reclaim her true identity, which always was and always will be much more than any label. I wish I had been able to read this book many years ago when I was a much younger therapist, ideally before I first met Sheila. The combination of solid, practical information and uplifting ideas in this book constitute an invaluable resource for health care professionals at all levels of experience.

Yvonne Dolan,
President of the Solution-Focused Brief Therapy Association

Acknowledgments

While preparing this book, our colleague, friend, and mentor, Steve de Shazer, died on September 11, 2005. Steve and his wife and partner, Insoo Kim Berg, were the original developers of the solution-focused brief approach. Joel once asked Steve whether he had ever envisioned that his ideas would have such an impact on the therapy field. Steve replied that this was something he never could have predicted, and that it came as a total surprise to him. He went on to say that he was not sure what he would have done had he not chosen to go in the direction of solution-focused practices, but speculated that he probably would have been tending bar somewhere. We are grateful to Steve and the influence that he has had on our thinking. Evidence of this influence is on every page and in every word of this book.

Joel wishes to extend a special acknowledgment to our colleague, Dan Gallagher, who has been Joel's mentor and solution-focus guide, and who often challenges Joel's thinking. We extend our appreciation to Yvonne Dolan who supported and encouraged this book. Gale Miller was kind enough to review and advise us on the chapter titled "Tools of Solution-Focused Brief Practice." We are indebted to Insoo Kim Berg who has been our teacher and guide.

Thorana would like to acknowledge her colleagues with the Solution-Focused Brief Therapy Association, where she met Joel and many other wonderful solution-focused people. She also wishes to acknowledge and thank her many students over the years, who have challenged and encouraged her to be clear in her thinking, and have rewarded her richly.

Finally, we give grateful acknowledgment to our solution-focused colleagues all over the world, and, most of all, to the clients with whom we have had the privilege of working. They have been the richest wellsprings of our learning.

Solution-Focused Brief Practice
© 2007 by The Haworth Press, Taylor & Francis Group. All rights reserved.
doi:10.1300/5507_b

Chapter 1

Introduction

In July 1988, Joel was offered a newly created position, Intensive Case Manager (ICM), with a local agency in Orange County, New York. New York State had initiated the ICM program to reduce the total inpatient hospitalizations among those who had been designated as seriously and persistently mentally ill (SPMI) by providing trained clinicians who, in effect, acted as ombudsmen for a limited caseload of clients[1] with high inpatient psychiatric admissions.

Orange County was one of a select number of counties in New York State chosen to test the ICM program. Joel was one of the first ICMs in New York and the first in Orange County. Selecting a suitable caseload was relatively simple: obtain a computer printout of the 10 highest inpatient recidivists in the local state psychiatric hospital and work with them. These were to be Joel's clients. He provided case management services, transportation, and direct clinical services when no other providers were involved.

Joel worked with his clients in their life spaces, often visiting them in their homes. Very often, individuals ancillary to the client also were involved with the mental health system[2] as caretakers. The major thrust of maintaining stability within the client's social system mandated that Joel also include these significant others in his work with the client. Joel had free access to the state psychiatric hospital, which allowed him to continue to work with clients who were hospitalized.

During the course of Joel's work with the clients, he came to know each one of them individually beyond their diagnoses and their roles as "mental health patients." In addition, working within the local mental health system, he gained insights into patterns of interventions that were helpful, and many that were not. The lessons learned in this position and subsequent positions led to insights that were re-

Solution-Focused Brief Practice
© 2007 by The Haworth Press, Taylor & Francis Group. All rights reserved.
doi:10.1300/5507_01

inforced when Joel finally came in contact with the ideas of solution-focused brief practice (SFBP)[3] in the early 1990s.

The first lesson—and probably the one that had the most impact—was that although these were clients with the highest number of annual hospitalizations, there were periods—some longer than others—when most people enjoyed relatively stable functioning. Joel quickly learned to suspend his role as expert and listen to what the clients had to say about what it was that helped them stay out of the hospital or helped them get discharged more quickly when they were hospitalized. The role of the ICM became much simpler: rather than dictate certain things as "best," Joel would find out what clients did that helped them stay out of the hospital, encourage them in these practices, and help them do more of them. The aim of the ICM was not to "cure," but (1) to help clients function as well as they possibly could, and (2) to minimize psychiatric hospitalizations.

Despite their long-term patient status and the expectations that accompany this status, many of the clients courageously and persistently maintained a sense that they were somehow more than their diagnoses or their patient status. One client was an inventor who had one invention highlighted in *Popular Mechanics* magazine. Another had been a jazz pianist who, when he had the opportunity to play, exhibited an amazing transformation from psychiatric patient to creative and competent artist. When asked, clients were able to talk about their interests, hopes, aspirations, internal and external resources, strengths, and competencies.

Dr. Gale Miller (personal communication, July 15, 1997), professor of sociology at Marquette University in Milwaukee, Wisconsin, reflected that doing SFBP requires the ability to notice the extraordinary things that individuals do in their ordinary lives. The clients that Joel worked with illustrate Miller's observation. Throughout their difficult lives, they somehow maintained courage and strength that helped them preserve a spark of hope for a better future and a sense of possibilities.

During the course of Joel's tenure as an ICM, he observed conversations that the clients had with mental health professionals. Contacts usually were brief and centered on whether the individual was "compliant" with the prescribed course of treatment. Clients often were admonished that they needed to take their medications and see their therapists regularly or suffer the risk of hospitalization.

Conversations with doctors focused on compliance, and physicians instructed clients that they had a disease similar to diabetes that needed to be managed. Clients who told their doctors about any future aspirations or hopes were advised that they needed to keep the amount of stress in their lives within manageable levels and therefore needed to have more realistic goals for the future. It was not surprising that for some clients, these conversations served to dampen their hopes and reinforce their beliefs of incompetence and hopelessness about themselves.

In a moving speech, Dr. Patricia Deegan (1993) reflected on her experiences as an adolescent when she was first diagnosed with major mental illness:

> I was thinking about my first couple of hospitalizations when I was first diagnosed with schizophrenia, and three months later, at my second hospital admission, I was labeled with chronic schizophrenia. I was told I had a disease that was like diabetes, and if I continued to take neuroleptic medications for the rest of my life and avoided stress, that I might be able to cope. (p. 2)

She continued, talking about the effect that this conversation had on her:

> And I remember that as these words were spoken to me by my psychiatrist, it felt as if my whole world began to crumble and shatter. My teenage world in which I aspired to dreams of being a valued person in valued roles—of playing lacrosse for the U.S. Women's Team or maybe joining the Peace Corps—I felt these parts of my identity being stripped from me. I felt myself beginning to undergo that radically dehumanizing and devaluing transformation from being a person to being an illness: from being Pat Deegan to being "a schizophrenic." (p. 2)

Other clients fought bravely against the "radically dehumanizing and devaluating transformation," and it is not surprising that those clients who struggled to maintain some modicum of self beyond their diagnoses stopped going to the clinic and avoided the conversations. They also had been prescribed medications that often had side effects such as stiffness, restlessness, and what clients usually identified as "a drugged out feeling" that limited their abilities to work, play, and love. The professionals then gave additional labels to clients who avoided treatment: noncompliant and resistant. When they did go to see their doctors or therapists, they were warned that if they continued avoiding treatment they would once again find themselves in the state hospital, all too often a self-fulfilling prophesy.

After his time as an ICM, Joel was hired as director of a community mental health clinic licensed by the New York State Office of Mental Health. Typical of such clinics, it served a wide range of clients, especially those from a lower socioeconomic stratum. In this new setting, Joel continued working with those clients who had been long-term users of the mental health system. As he incorporated the solution-focused approach in his practice as both a supervisor and clinician, he once again became interested and curious about what individuals do on a day-to-day basis that helps them live satisfying lives.

Joel's next experience was as a treatment coordinator for a private psychiatric hospital, which provided him additional insights into the effects of the medical model within a psychiatric system. Despite the often frustrating sense that the application of the medical model to clinical treatment is akin to fitting the proverbial square peg into a round hole, the actual day-to-day solution-focused work with clients afforded additional evidence that SFBP provides a set of tools that can be very effectively applied to working with clients within a psychiatric system. This book is about how we can better listen to clients, and in so doing, learn how to co-construct more useful conversations about clients' goals, resources, strengths, and possibilities.

One of the most difficult tasks we faced in writing this book was how we would refer to the individuals about whom we are writing. Two major considerations needed to be made: The first is the lesson we have learned (whether as clinicians, ICMs, clinic directors, SFBP trainers, or university professors) that no matter what the label, it can serve only to limit our ability to experience another individual holistically; labels are reductionistic and necessarily omit much information. Metaphorically, they are only snapshots of an individual's behavior at a specific time in a specific place. The second consideration regards the scope of the topic. Long-term users of the mental health system do not include just those who are psychiatrically diagnosed, but those who have permanent physical challenges as well and who frequently utilize the services of mental health professionals.

Many clinicians seem to believe that SFBP is not appropriate for "real," "hard," or "serious" situations. They especially seem to believe that SFBP cannot be helpful for situations that include behaviors, symptoms, and diagnoses that are considered permanent or incurable. These people often are called "chronic users" of services and are unable to benefit from therapy except for "managing" their "illnesses." We prefer to think of them as people—people who may have biological, physiological, or psychological conditions that limit their abilities to function as well as many other people, but people who most likely have more potential than most would think. We believe that SFBP is uniquely helpful to those clients who may need intermittent support for long periods or for most of their lives, and who are more than their diagnosis. Thus, we refer to these clients as long-term users of services rather than as chronically mentally ill or something else. These clients may need frequent or infrequent services, for very short or longer periods in each occurrence, and for very short or longer sessions of conversation.

Joel recalls one of his clients who, after years of therapy and several diagnoses, declared that he realized one day that he was more than his label. We thought that this was an especially good starting point for the book and, in its simplest and most elegant form, why we thought that it was time for a book about solution-focused work with long-term users of the mental health system. Our review of the applicable literature highlighted the paucity of information regarding the application of SFBP to individuals who too often become victims of a system that confers labels that serve to limit their possibilities.

This book holds in common with solution-focused literature the general principle of finding out what works and doing more of it. In this regard, it would be appropriate to conclude our introduction with an applicable quote from Dr. Deegan:

> You see, I would argue that until the fundamental relationship between people who have been psychiatrically labeled and those who have not changes, until the radical power imbalance between us is at least equalized, until our relationships are marked by true mutuality, and until we recognize the common ground of our shared humanity and stop the spirit-breaking effects of dehumanization in the mental health system, then that gaping hole will continue to sink the best of our efforts. (1993, p. 2)

We write this book for those clinicians and clients who are able to see beyond psychiatric labels, beyond symptoms and limitations, and beyond the limitations of those who assign labels into futures of possibilities and hope for better lives.

The purpose of the book is to provide students and providers who may not be conversant with solution-focused ideas an opportunity to understand and explore this very different way of working with those who may be considered as suffering from severe or chronic psychological problems or mental illnesses. Readers of Chapter 2 will enjoy definitions and descriptions of the basic assumptions, concepts, and practices of the approach. Subsequent chapters will illustrate ideas for working with clients who were diagnosed with various mental illnesses and who have long histories of psychiatric treatment. Three chapters describe first the ways that SFBP is different from a medical model for understanding the problems people bring to us, views from four psychiatrists who use SFBP in their practices, and ways that solution-focused perspectives can be helpful for establishing SFB practices in agencies and hospitals. We conclude with a chapter on the philosophies that guide our thinking about SFBP.

NOTES

1. We use the term *client* in this book to denote a professional and contractual relationship between a user of mental health services and a provider.

2. It seems contradictory to the authors to call something mental *health* when the system focuses on mental *illness*. However, for the sake of convention, we use the term *mental health*.

3. The original solution-focused work was centered on therapy. Today, solution-focused ideas are used in a variety of contexts, including social services, corrections, and even business. Steve de Shazer suggested the concept of solution-focused brief practice. Therefore, we use the acronym SFBP.

Chapter 2

Tools of Solution-Focused
Brief Practice

The solution-focused brief practice approach is, above all, an approach, a stance, or a perspective. It is not a Theory of how people develop, how people change, or how therapy should be conducted. One could say, we suppose, that "one theory" (note the small *t*) is that a solution-focused approach in therapy helps clients make the changes they wish to make because they focus on what they want rather than on what they do not want. This is as far as the approach goes, in terms of theory, however. In Chapter 9, the philosophies that inform our understanding of the approach will be explained in terms of post-structuralism, social constructionism, and language games. In this chapter we describe some of the basic elements of the SFBP stance: assumptions, concepts, and practices.

STANCE

During the 2002 European Brief Therapy Association conference in Cardiff, Wales, a question was asked: "When did you realize that you became solution-focused?" Joel's response was that he had originally learned to ask questions to which he would probably know the answer. SFBP takes a very different stance: practitioners ask questions only the client can answer. Joel answered that he became solution-focused when his questions became driven by his curiosity about clients' responses.

One of the chief elements of SFBP is a stance of *curiosity*. That is, the therapist does not "know" what is happening with the client or what course of action clients should take to better their circum-

Solution-Focused Brief Practice
doi:10.1300/5507_02

stances. When a client says he or she is "bipolar," or a referring person states that the client is "schizophrenic," the SFB therapist does not pretend to know what this means in the particular situation. The *Diagnostic and Statistical Manual of Mental Disorders* (DSM-IV; American Psychiatric Association, 1994) lists criteria for various diagnoses; these criteria are not *all* present, however, in every case. Neither are they present *all* of the time or with the same severity all of the time. Also, these behaviors are not the only behaviors or characteristics of the client.

Finally, no two situations have the exact same contextual factors. No two people have the same family, friends, work or school situation, resources, or stressors. Especially, no two people *experience* these contextual and cultural factors, their own characteristics, their symptoms, or the interactions of people around them in the same way. Therefore, it is important for the therapist to be curious about the client's unique situation.

Similarly, no two people or situations will require or find suitable the same solutions. What works for one person or family in one situation/context may or may not be helpful to another situation or person. Therefore, again, the SFB therapist maintains a sense of profound curiosity about what will be helpful to each unique client.

The SFB therapist does not maintain a stance of diagnosing, hypothesizing, or attempting to discover underlying causes or dysfunctions related to the symptom. This *nonpathologizing* aspect of the SFBP stance is very important. Using DSM criteria to diagnose and then develop treatment plans based on theoretical underlying problems and treatments is not helpful in this work. Maintaining an abiding faith in the nonpathology of all persons is very important. It is tempting for those trained in traditional psychotherapeutic models to "see" all sorts of things that are wrong with clients; this is second nature to good training. So when a client comes for help and talks about voices that the therapist does not hear, the SFB therapist does not get caught up in concerns about what is "really" going on with the client or about particular solutions such as medication. Rather, the stances of curiosity and nonpathologizing lead the therapist to wonder about how this particular client experiences the voices, to try to understand how this situation is a problem and for whom, and to explore a wide range of ideas around goals and ways to meet those goals in therapy.

A corollary to the nonpathologizing stance is one of not having preconceived ideas about so-called *normal* behavior. For any person in any context, what seems unusual to some people may and most likely does make total sense to the client. Active children with teachers who are concerned that they have ADHD (attention-deficit/hyperactivity disorder) or a similar disability may be responding to all sorts of possibilities, including the chance that the child's nervous system is different from that of children who are more able to sit still. However, a range of behavior exists in such situations, as does a range of ideas about what is acceptable or tolerable. The perspectives developed through language and social consensus have as much to do with what gets identified as problematic as does anything else. The child's active behavior may not be problematic on the playground or at home or even at school with other teachers. In fact, it is most likely that the child's behavior is not problematic at all times or with the same severity, and in some contexts may actually be a resource.

SFB therapists approach each situation and each session *tentatively*. Because it is not possible to know what is going on completely or even to understand the client's perspective fully, it is important to go gently into each conversation, carefully attending to what the clients are saying in their own language, and holding our own ideas very cautiously. Our ideas are based on our own experiences, not the clients', so we must be careful how we use those experiences.

Through these stances the therapist demonstrates profound *respect* for the client. Clients must respect therapists in order for the therapists to be helpful to them. Respect is earned, chiefly by being very respectful of clients and their experiences. Believing that we are somehow more knowledgeable about clients' lives is not a helpful stance for solution-building. Clients may respect therapists who act as experts because of socially learned respect for authority and because they feel they need help; however, in the SFBP approach, therapists take a "not-knowing stance" (Anderson & Goolishian, 1992), and therefore must genuinely trust and respect that clients know what is best for their situations.

ASSUMPTIONS AND CONCEPTS

The first important assumption of SFBP is that the only constant is change. Nothing stays the same and nothing is the same or means the same thing in all situations. Lashing out at someone may be problematic in one context but appropriate in another, for example. The expression of anger is different in each situation.

SFB therapists capitalize on this idea that change is inevitable and use it to the advantage of the clients' situations. One simple example is when clients report small improvements or small differences from one time to another. This small change exemplifies that change can happen, and the therapist uses this to help clients increase hope and see progress toward therapeutic goals. Clients usually come to therapists because they perceive that a problem is constant and unchanging and that they have no solutions left to try on their own. This is an illusion, and part of the therapist's job is to help the client deconstruct the constancy of the problem.

Related to the idea that change is always happening is the idea that small changes lead to larger changes. Many therapeutic approaches use numerous sessions of therapy to help clients reach goals, and discourage finishing therapy until all goals are fully reached. Because the SFB therapist believes that change happens and that small changes lead to larger changes, similar to ripple or domino effects, therapy may need only to get things moving in a helpful direction. Clients often can continue moving toward their goals on their own once therapy has helped them find a good direction and tools that work.

This idea is especially important for working with clients for whom a "serious" diagnosis has been made or who will always experience life in ways that are problematic for them and/or for others. By focusing on change, on goals, and on the idea that one meaningful change leads to another, clients remain hopeful about their situations, whether this means that their symptoms go away or that they are more able to enjoy life in spite of the difficulties. Feeling competent rather than not-competent, these clients may be more able to manage their lives because of the trust and faith in them demonstrated by their therapists. This also may make it easier for clients to return to therapy when circumstances require, trusting that they have not gone back to "square one" but have just hit a bump in the road and that change can happen again for them. In fact, one common question asked by solution-focused practitioners when clients return to therapy is, "What did you forget to do that you did last time to get yourself on track?"

The ideas that change happens and that small changes lead to larger changes point toward other assumptions of SFBP: clients are unique, they are the best experts on their own lives, they have strengths and resources for solving their problems, and therapy is most helpful when client competency is co-constructed. As discussed earlier, no two clients or situations are the same, even when the labels used to describe them are the same. They are the only ones who can describe their experiences, and they generally have more competence than many traditional therapists are able to see, often because the therapists see the client through the cloak of their preferred theories. Therapists who use theories based on problem solving usually look more for what is not working than for what *is* working for the client. One of the unfortunate effects of labels is that therapists begin to believe the labels or the characteristics they exemplify are the essence, the core of a person. This clouds the therapist's vision for strengths and resources possessed by the client and leads to giving advice or prescribing certain treatments.

Similarly, no two clients will respond to treatment in the same way and, when treatment seems to fail, therapists often blame clients for being "resistant." de Shazer declared the "death of resistance" in 1984, pointing out that clients who seem resistant are telling us how they cooperate with us. Treatments, advice, or homework assignments may or may not be helpful to a particular client, and one of the therapist's jobs is to discover how the client is cooperating and use this feedback to adjust the therapy so that it is useful to the client. In this view, the client is not resisting therapy; instead, therapy may not have a good enough fit for the client. In the SFBP approach, it is not useful to blame clients for apparent failures, but to use the opportunity to learn more about the client's unique circumstance to find fitting solutions.

By definition, problems imply solutions. Something that cannot change, such as a disability, is life (I. K. Berg, personal communication, July, 1997), a situation, not a problem. The client and therapist together may be able to help the client find better ways to cope with the situation or to overcome its effects. Attempting to change unchangeable situations is doomed to failure.

Also, it is important to remember that some things do not need changing or managing. "If it ain't broke, don't fix it! Once you know what works, do more of it! If it doesn't work, then don't do it again— do something different!" (Berg & Miller, 1992, p. 17). Often, attempts to find solutions result in making the situation worse (Watzlawick,

Weakland, & Fisch, 1974). In those situations, the solution becomes the problem, and a new solution must be developed, one that may not seem related to the original problem. Similarly, the therapist and client may discover that what the client or others thought was the problem was not the problem at all. In a video (de Shazer, 1985), de Shazer helped a client realize that she suffered from a sleep problem, not difficulties with the man in the upstairs apartment. She believed that the man was beaming something through the ceiling, and that this was the cause of her worrying, which kept her awake at night. The usual practice would be to define this problem as delusional. de Shazer and the woman together co-constructed it as a sleep problem. Once she and de Shazer began exploring exceptions to the sleep problem and exploring alternative ways of making sure she had a good night's sleep, the problem with the man upstairs disappeared.

PRACTICES

In this section, we describe common practices in the solution-focused approach. We hesitate to use the words *techniques* or *interventions,* because those words often connote an idea that the therapist does something *to* the client. The SFBP approach focuses on collaborative conversations between clients and therapists rather than therapists' doing something to clients. We recognize, however, that therapists in the SFBP approach are trained, supervised, and experienced in particular kinds of conversations—ones that build solutions rather than exploring problems. Therefore, obviously SFB therapists use specific interventions. We call these *practices* or *tools.*

Goals

One of the most important aspects of the SFBP approach is its focus on client goals. Most therapies focus on goals, but these goals often are related to Theory (e.g., individuation, stronger boundaries, or changing distorted thoughts) and the absence of the problems or symptoms. These kinds of goals may be reached as part of therapy, but they are not the therapist's focus or target. Rather, goals are developed from the *client's* desires, not the therapist's or theory's. Well-formed goals guide the conversation and help the therapist and client know when therapy is ready to be ended. Goals (1) are important to the client; (2) are placed in relational contexts; (3) are the presence of something wanted rather than the absence of something unwanted; (4) emphasize beginnings of change, not necessarily the end points; (5) are concrete, realistic, and measurable; and (6) involve roles for each client.

Throughout our discussion of different practices, it is important to keep in mind that SFBP arose from interactional therapies, including Milton Erickson and the Mental Research Institute (MRI) approach (Watzlawick et al., 1974). Although many SFBP practices focus on individuals and their thinking, as will be evident, thinking always occurs in a relational context, even when only one client is in the client-therapist relationship. Therapists keep in mind that clients also live in relational contexts with other people who are affected by and who affect the clients' lives. These people, even when not present in therapy, are part of a client's system and are a rich resource for solution-building.

It is easy in therapy to focus on eliminating symptoms as the goal. However, doing this keeps the focus on the problems and tempts clients and therapists to discuss the nature of the problem, the effects of the problem, the causes of the problem, and so forth. Focusing attention with clients on problems serves to co-construct problems even more and expecting solutions to magically emerge from such conversations is not realistic. The talk must shift from problems to solutions for this to occur.

For some clients, problem talk seems more important than for others. However, the SFBP approach turns therapy on its head and focuses on what will be different when the problem is gone, and ways for the client to make that happen. "Going for walks in the woods" is easier for clients to imagine and to do than is "staying away from alcohol, which isn't good for me." In many ways, discussions about goals serve to invite clients into solution-building conversations. One hallmark of SFBP is looking to the future rather than the past as a way of reaching goals more easily. SFBP is also action-oriented and therapy helps clients to imagine and then do the things needed to reach their goals. It is not necessary to focus on problems to do this.

Similarly, because two of the assumptions of SFBP are that change happens and that small changes lead to bigger changes, therapy focuses on the smallest change necessary to help the client begin moving in the desired direction. It is easy to understand how thinking ahead to a long-off time when the problem is eliminated leads to feelings of defeat and being overwhelmed. By focusing on the first step, or the first small change possible, clients are encouraged to begin changes carefully. In some ways, this is important so that wrong steps are recognized quickly. In other ways, this practice builds hope, a sense of competence and accomplishment, and makes the goals seem more possible.

Clients do not need to reach their stated goals to end therapy; once they are on track and express confidence in their abilities to stay on track (or get back on track if there's a slip), they may wish to end therapy. Goals are not fixed but remain fluid. The reasons that clients decide that they no longer need therapy are often minimally or not at all related to the original goal. SFB therapists do not have a need for clients to fully reach their goals in order to terminate therapy. Of course, clients may wish to return for booster sessions some time in the future if they feel stuck. This often is true of those who have been long-term users of mental health services. Many clients, however, need only to remind themselves of the solution-building conversations to get going again.

Clients sometimes present to therapy with vague goals. When possible, it is good to develop an understanding of details and the contexts of goals. A number of questions can help clients determine concrete signs of reaching goals: "How will you know that it's okay to finish therapy?" or "What will your spouse see that will tell her that you're closer to your goals?"

On the other hand, some goals are very difficult for clients to determine in specific ways. "I don't know" is one of the most frustrating things that clients can say to us, and some therapists see that response as evasive or as displaying resistance. One of the rules of most language games is "turn taking." In any given conversation, it is expected that each party takes turns—one talks, the other responds, and so forth. Imagine our reaction if we said something to someone and received no response. SFB practitioners understand "I don't know" as the client's attempt to follow the social rules. Our first reaction when the client says "I don't know" is to wait and give the client time to think. Again following social rules that forbid silence, and given time, most clients respond with something.

However, sometimes, clients really do not know what will be different. In those situations, scales can provide concrete measures for change. The scaling numbers become the concrete markers, even though the meanings of the points on the scale may change (see the following section on scaling questions).

Whenever possible, clients' relational contexts should be included as part of therapy. Systemic change is more likely to be long-lasting and satisfying to clients and the people around them. This is true for so-called "individual" problems as well as more obviously relational problems such as couples or family difficulties. In addition to being curious as to how others would identify important changes, these people also are resources for each other. Thinking about what a caring other person might notice places that person more clearly in the client's context and may then be noticed as a resource. In the broadest sense, the job of the SFBP is to initiate and foster solution-building conversations. Asking about the client's social contexts serves to continue the process of solution-building in those contexts.

Exceptions

Problems are not happening all the time or all the time with the same intensity. Looking for exceptions helps clients reduce the cloud of doom that tends to form, pushing clients into therapy. By the time clients reach us, they often have tried "everything" to ameliorate the problem and literally are at their wits' end. That is, they are not able to think of anything new to try. By noticing times when the problem is not present or is not problematic, or times when it is less noticeable, clients are able to begin to notice resources and strengths that they may not have known they had, may not have remembered, or may not have thought of as possibilities for helping with the current situation. Similarly, noticing times when the problem would be expected, but is not present, also helps clients and therapists enlarge the picture of possibilities, and to find both old (but forgotten) and new solutions. We have learned from our clients that exceptions often are not differences that make a difference (Bateson, 1972) within a problem-focused language game. On the other hand, when clients accept our invitations into solution-building, the same exceptions appear to make a difference.

Presuppositional Questions

Pressupositional questions are similar to exceptions. By presupposing that the problem is not always present or problematic, the ther-

apist helps the client develop a future picture in which the problem is
not present or is less problematic. If something is available in the
present or the recent past, it is likely that the client will be able to project it into the future. Presuppositional questions are open. That is, a
presuppositional question might be, "What do you see that is green?"
This question assumes that something green is present. On the other
hand, if the therapist asks, "Is there something green?" the client is more
likely to say no without fully scanning the context. Presuppositional
questions include asking about presession change, such as, "What is
better about your problem since the time you made the appointment
to come here?" or "What will your sister notice is different when you
have reached your goal half way?" (Weiner-Davis, de Shazer, &
Gingerich, 1987).

The Miracle Question

The *miracle question* (MQ; Berg & Miller, 1992) has become almost synonymous with SFBP. The MQ asks people to imagine that
after the therapy appointment, they go home, finish their day as they
usually do, go to sleep, and while they are asleep a miracle happens,
and the problems that brought them to therapy are gone, just like *that*.
But, because they were asleep, they did not know the miracle happened. Then the therapist asks, "What is the first thing you would
notice upon awakening that would tell you that a miracle had happened?"

Asking the MQ helps the client and the therapist identify goals for
therapy. "What will be happening when the voices are not bothering
you so much that you cannot go to work? What's the first thing you
will notice?" This helps the client and therapist to identify concrete
goals. In this example, the client might identify getting up in the morning and fixing breakfast. Obviously, these are actions easier to plan
and take than "stopping the voices." Fixing breakfast might be the
first small and meaningful step on a new road toward a time when the
problem is not happening, is not problematic, or is less problematic.

Sometimes clients identify something that is not possible; winning
the lottery or having a deceased loved one back are common responses.
In these cases, the therapist might smile and nod empathically, but
say nothing. Clients know when impossible things are impossible.
Soon, they typically respond with something more realistic.

Follow-up questions to the MQ are very important. We have heard many therapists say that they asked the MQ, but it "didn't work." We have never had this experience, because the MQ is not designed to suddenly make goals and solutions appear. Rather, it is part of a solution-building conversation that helps clients and therapists move along the track toward goals. Follow-up questions include, "What else?" "How could you make that happen?" and "What difference might that make in your life?" Finding out what differences do for a person or system (differences that make differences; Bateson, 1972) helps the client and therapist enlarge the picture of possibilities and notice other things that might make a difference.

For example, if fixing breakfast might make a difference in terms of eating better, it might be useful to find out what "eating better" means to the client. It is important for therapists to not assume that they know what something means. In this case, "eating better" could be related to nutrition, to socializing with the family, to starting the day "right," or to all sorts of possible things. It also is important that a therapist not assume that a difference is too small. The meaningfulness of the difference is for the client to judge. The therapist's job is to co-construct useful meanings of the differences by asking details of how the change will make a difference to the client and to those in the client's life.

Additional follow-up questions to the MQ include relational questions (De Jong & Berg, 2002). These questions enlarge the client's context by bringing important others into it. For example, what would a spouse notice that would tell him or her that a miracle had occurred? Supposing the first thing a client noticed was that she or he would feel like getting out of bed. "What difference would that make to someone else in the house?" "What else?" ("What else?" is a question that can be used in many places and many times. Therapists may begin to think that they sound like broken records—however, it is amazing how much "What else?" does to help clients build solutions.) Some clients claim that no one would notice because no one else is present or because no one else cares. Rather than arguing, it sometimes is useful to ask what that person would notice if she or he did care or was present. Or, what would the cat notice? A dog would notice that its owner was taking it for more walks.

Exceptions also are useful to notice as part of the MQ practice. It is common for SFB therapists to ask about the last time even a little bit of the miracle occurred, and to follow this up with relational or other questions. It is important to ask about details in these situations. Creating a picture that is as full of detail as possible helps to enlarge the picture, make more possibilities noticeable, and provide clues for small steps the client can take toward the miracle.

Scaling Questions

Scaling questions are not unique to SFBP, but are used extensively, creatively, and positively. Motivational interviewing (MI; Cordova, Warren, & Gee, 2001) is similar to SFBP scaling in that clients are asked to rate themselves on a scale of 1 to 10 on some factor such as progress toward a goal. The difference between SFBP scaling and MI is one of perspective. Let us say that the client responds with "two," 10 being the best possible. In MI, the therapist would be worried that the client is far from the goal, noticing that much work needs to be done. The SFBP therapist would notice that 2 is better than 0 or 1 and wonder what makes it so high. Yes, it is a long way from the goal, but it is somewhere, not nowhere. We can also be curious with the client about which pieces of that 10 are happening at 2.

Beginning practitioners of SFBT frequently make the mistake of seeing the numbers as concrete and real. They become disappointed when a client states she or he is at a 2 on the scale. We learn through experience that the numbers in and of themselves have no meaning until the client and therapist make meaning together through solution-building conversations.

Joel recalls having one client who said that he was lower than 0 on a 0 to 10 scale. Joel changed the scale to –5 to +5. The client then answered that he was at a –3. Of course, Joel became curious why he was not –4 or –5.

A frequent next step for using scaling is to ask what one or one-half step up the scale would look like or where on the scale the client needs to be to say that therapy is over. Relational questions also are useful in conjunction with scaling questions. For example, what would some important other notice that would tell him or her that the client had moved one step closer to the goal? What would tell the client that this person (or pet) had noticed? These questions help to solidify possibilities and make the client and others alert to noticing their presence. That is, if the client actually is doing *x*, which is one step closer to the goal, does that not mean that the client *is* one step closer? Noticing these small changes helps to instill hope, courage, and satisfaction with the therapy process.

Some people like to use the numbers on the scale to quantify change. We are mindful, however, that what seems like a 3 one week may be a 7 another week. Similarly, even though a client is doing the things he or she said would mean a 6, that client might decide, when reaching that goal, that it really is an 8. This fluid way of thinking helps therapists be very creative in the use of scaling. A client, when asked where things were in a second session, replied, "negative ten." It would be easy for the therapist to become discouraged with such an answer. However, the therapist could ask questions such as, "What keeps it from being a negative twenty?" or "How have you managed to cope with such a bad week/day/life?"

Coping Questions

Coping questions are useful, as described previously, when the client is very discouraged and seems unable to envision a future that is different from the miserable past. Responses to coping questions shore the client up as a person who has strengths and abilities, if only to cope and to keep things from being absolutely worse. The therapist can follow up with questions about what difference it makes when the client is coping even a little, what difference it makes to others, what those people notice that tells them the client is coping, what coping a little better would look like, and so forth. We often find that coping questions paradoxically help us and the client move from discouragement and despair to hope and solution-building.

Other SFBP practices include taking a *break* near the end of the session, giving *compliments,* and offering *messages* and *suggestions* or *experiments* that the client might wish to try after the session. The session break evolved through the use of observing teams in therapy. The therapist would take a short break to consult with a team of co-workers who had been observing the session from behind a one-way mirror. The therapist and the team would discuss the session and devise ideas to communicate to the client. These ideas often would serve as a bridge between what happened during the session and the suggested task (De Jong & Berg, 2002). The post-break message includes compliments that the team offers that are based on things they heard from the client. These are then used as a frame for the suggestion. For example, the team might compliment the client on her ability to be so articulate about how the voices were affecting her, which is particularly remarkable given that she says the voices make her confused. Because she is so articulate, the team would like her to try an experiment: notice the times when she is able to be articulate in spite of the voices.

Notice that the goal, or at least the initial goal, is not to make the voices disappear but to diminish their effects in the client's life. These practices, when combined into a whole, similar to a painting that is in progress, help the client and the therapist notice much more in the life of the client than just the problems. By comparison, problems fade in the client's life, and other things that may have always been there, at least in terms of potential, become clearer. Focusing on problems tends to make them more prominent than exceptions; focusing on exceptions to problems, to resources and strengths, and to solutions diminishes the problems.

CONCLUSION

In this chapter, our purpose was to present the basic tenets of SFBP. It is very often tempting in clinical practice to treat ideas as Theories. It should be remembered that SFBP began as an inductive approach in which the developers (and those of us who have followed) learned what works directly from our clients. This requires the ability to listen to clients unencumbered by theoretical constructs that may otherwise constrain our vision. Presession change questions, the miracle question, scaling questions, exception questions, and coping questions are useful tools that have been developed by listening to clients and have been proven by the test of time and practice. This does not mean that each one will work all of the time with all clients. It is useful to have many tools in the toolbox so that if one does not work the way the clinician hopes, another one may.

Chapter 3

Mary "The Borderline"

The DSM-IV (APA, 1994) attempts to categorize psychosocial, pathological conditions by using neutral behavioral descriptions. The intention is to objectively and scientifically group and codify behavior. Yet, "objective science" becomes illusory when nothing strikes more fear in the collective hearts of most therapists than the dreaded (allegedly neutral) diagnosis of "borderline personality disorder."

In his article, *On Being Sane in Insane Places,* Rosenhan (1973) stated:

> Based in part on theoretical and anthropological considerations, but also on philosophical, legal, and therapeutic ones, the view has grown that psychological categorization of mental illness is useless at best and downright harmful, misleading and pejorative at worst. Psychiatric diagnoses, in this view, are in the minds of the observers and are not valid summaries of characteristics displayed by the observed. (p. 250)

Simon and Berg (2004) echoed this sentiment:

> Insurance companies require diagnoses and licensing bodies expect professionals to provide relevant assessment information to proper requests. Accordingly, solution-focused therapists comply with such requirements. . . . Beyond what third-party payers require, solution-focused therapists find little relevance or usefulness in diagnosis. (p. 140)

Diagnoses have powerful effects on clients' views of themselves and thus on their futures. Although diagnoses can be comforting by helping clients feel not alone and by giving names to seemingly unex-

Solution-Focused Brief Practice
© 2007 by The Haworth Press, Taylor & Francis Group. All rights reserved.
doi:10.1300/5507_03

plainable phenomena, Rosenhan (1973) stated that diagnoses act as self-fulfilling prophecies: "Eventually, the patient himself [sic] accepts the diagnosis, with all of its surplus meanings and expectations and behaves accordingly" (p. 256). That is, in addition to possibly explaining some symptoms, a diagnosis carries with it an assumption that a person so diagnosed most likely has all or most of the listed symptoms and may in fact develop these "surpluses" *after* receiving the diagnosis. In addition, once diagnosed, such people often are assumed to have not only a laundry list of symptoms, but also very limited capabilities beyond the diagnosed category.

Booker and Blymyer (1994) shared this point of view: "The traditional focus on pathology reinforces this clinical helplessness and reinforces the assumption that the client will need long-term treatment; psychotropic medication; and, all too often, psychiatric hospitalizations for extended periods of time" (p. 63).

Finally, Thomas Szasz (1970) expressed an even stronger view: "Like the inquisitor, the psychiatrist can 'sentence' a person to mental illness, but cannot wipe out the stigma he himself [sic] has imposed. In psychiatry, moreover, there is no pope to grant absolute pardon from a publicly affirmed diagnosis of mental illness" (p. 56).

Diagnosis can have a similar impact on the therapist who constructs realities about the client even before the first contact. Before the first session even begins, the therapist, knowing the diagnosis, already views the client through the lens of assumptions and diagnoses (labels) that carry many, often negative assumptions about the person receiving treatment. We often have said that diagnoses say as much about the person doing the diagnosing as about the person being described. We find this especially true of the diagnosis of "borderline personality disorder" for which treatment is paradoxically expected to be unending and, at the same time, futile.

I'M A BORDERLINE, YOU KNOW

Mary[1] had been in the mental health system for many years. Her psychiatric history was replete with multiple hospitalizations and failed therapies. In fact, most local mental health professionals knew Mary, and, upon hearing her name, would most likely comment, "Oh, her—she's a real borderline."

Most of Mary's frequent hospitalizations occurred after she superficially cut her arms, a behavior in which she often engaged over the years, raising both the consternation and anxiety of the numerous mental illness professionals and the mobile mental health unit who had often intervened in her episodes. Mary had been treated and subsequently discharged from most of the community mental health clinics and day treatment programs in the county. She was referred to as noncompliant, highly resistive and, at times, downright violent in addition to her diagnosis, which was damning enough.

Mary was 34 years old and lived alone, supported by her monthly Social Security disability check, which she received because her psychiatric disability precluded gainful employment. County Child Protective Services (CPS) had placed her six-year-old daughter in foster care after Mary was found to be neglectful. The family court judge had granted Mary supervised biweekly visitations with her daughter.

According to the supervising agency's report, the visitations had not gone well; the daughter appeared to be distant from her mother and Mary often argued with the supervising worker. After discussion between the various agencies involved in Mary's and her daughter's lives, the county foster care agency recommended to family court that Mary be forced to concede her parental rights and place the child for adoption.

Despite the difficulties, Mary had assiduously attended the scheduled visitations with her daughter and had been compliant with the court's requirements in order to regain custody of the child. As seems frequent in such situations, as soon as Mary jumped through the prescribed metaphorical hoops, she was assigned others. She readily expressed her anger at having fulfilled the requirements and then having new ones added. In accord with the expectations and assumptions of her diagnosis, this behavior was defined as "splitting" and served to reinforce the view of Mary as "borderline."

Just prior to her treatment at the community mental health clinic supervised by Joel, Mary had attended an adult day treatment program daily. While there, she exhibited the same behaviors that marked her short tenures at other programs. She frequently expressed her anger to the other clients and especially to staff. There were times that her rage seemed to be uncontrollable and she had to be physically restrained from hurting others in the program.

Mary's attendance was sporadic and, after she again cut herself, the program director of the day treatment program explained to Mary that she could no longer attend the program. The director recommended that she continue her therapy at the clinic supervised by Joel—if not the last, certainly one of the last options left for her in the county.

The therapist, Andy Taylor, saw Mary, using a one-way mirror with a consulting team that included Joel. Almost immediately Mary informed Andy: "You know, I'm a borderline." Andy responded by asking Mary what she wanted to be different. Mary responded by expressing her anger at the caseworker, family court, and CPS in general. She acknowledged that she had not been the best possible mother, but insisted that she loved her child and had been working to accomplish whatever requirements were mandated by the court.

She had successfully completed a series of parenting classes, had faithfully attended every supervised visit with her daughter, and was attending therapy as ordered by the court. Mary described how her relationship with her daughter had recently improved: the daughter was more bonded to her and appeared to enjoy the relationship during their visits.

Mary said that the relationship was improving despite the limited contact and the difficulties imposed by having an observing third party present. She complained that the supervising worker did not seem to notice the improvements and instead focused on disagreements between her and her daughter. Mary also reported that she had found an alternative living arrangement that would be a more suitable situation for the eventual return of the daughter, although it placed greater burdens on her limited financial resources.

Mary stated that she needed to use therapy to express and "vent" her feelings about the unfair system that was keeping her from her daughter. When Andy asked her how such venting would be helpful to her, Mary replied that she was uncertain but that she was sure it would make her feel better at least for the moment. This was most likely how she understood the process of therapy, having been socialized by her many previous therapists. Andy spent a good portion of the first session with Mary trying to determine how an exploration of the difficulties she had had in the past and continued to experience might be helpful for the future.

Andy took the break and, after consulting with the team, returned to compliment Mary on the hard work that she had been doing in order to regain custody of her child. The team acknowledged that despite all of the hurdles that were being placed in front of her, Mary never wavered from her goal. The team members said to Mary that they could understand her anger regarding having fulfilled requirements only to have new ones added. They told Mary that it must be very hard and therefore admirable that Mary persevered despite her discouragement and frustration. The team could only guess how much Mary must really care for her daughter. Finally, the team acknowledged the progress that Mary was making with her daughter and noted that obviously her determination was paying off. All of these things were genuinely perceived by the team.

Andy told Mary that the team had had a long discussion about her conception of therapy and whether it was ultimately going to be helpful toward achieving her goal. Andy continued, saying that despite the team's concern about Mary's proposed methodology, they were willing to give it a try as long as it resulted in a positive difference.

Mary seemed pleased with the team's compliments and said that her hard work and perseverance had never been acknowledged before. Andy asked when she wanted to see the team and him again, and she replied that she would like an appointment in one week. The next week, she returned and complained about CPS, family court, her previous therapists, the psychiatric hospitals where she had been treated in the past, and the supervised visitations. Andy's attempts to invite Mary into a solution-building conversation were met with minimal responses, following which Mary continued to rail against past, present, and future purveyors of her trials and tribulations. The team once again acknowledged Mary's anger and complimented her on her perseverance. They again questioned whether they were being helpful, because it seemed that not much had changed during the prior week.

After each of the next three sessions, the team recommended to Mary that she notice the small signs that suggested to her that therapy was helping her achieve her goal. Mary returned each time, detailing the problems that she had experienced during the previous week. Andy attempted to engage her in a different language game,[2] but she responded minimally and continued her tirade. Each time, the team complimented her perseverance and questioned whether therapy was being helpful.

What Do You Want To Be Different?

In the fourth session, Mary reported to Andy that out of frustration and anger she had superficially scratched her arm with a razor the evening before and then made her way to the local mental health unit. Her wounds were cleansed and dressed, she was evaluated, and, because she did not seem to be immediately at risk for harm, the hospital sent her home, encouraging her to keep her therapy appointment the next day. Andy consulted the team at the end of the session. The discussion with the team centered on the apparent lack of progress in therapy, and the team questioned the advisability and ethics of continuing in a process that did not seem to bear fruit.

Andy returned to the therapy room to tell Mary the consensus of the team. He stated that engagement in problem talk is not something that appeared to be useful to Mary because she did not seem to be making much progress. Andy continued that he and the team agreed that it did not seem to make sense to continue something that was not being particularly useful and, given her actions of the previous evening, may in fact be making things worse.

Andy told Mary that the he was willing to continue to work with her but that he wanted to engage her in a very different conversation about her progress and strengths rather than her difficulties and weaknesses. Finally, Andy said to Mary that if she insisted that she wanted to continue in problem talk, he would be willing to help her find an alternative therapist.

At this, Mary stood up, very loudly screamed several expletives at Andy, pulled the door open with enough force to cause the clock on the team's side of the mirror to tumble to the floor, and walked out of the clinic. Luckily, the door hit a doorstop or else the doorknob would surely have shattered the one-way mirror.

The team members held a long discussion about their obligation and what action, if any, should be taken. It was clear that Mary knew the mental health system, knew how to call mobile mental health, and, if necessary, knew how to go to the hospital for physical treatment and evaluation. The team—albeit nervously—decided to take no action and to wait. Later that day, Mary called Andy and stated that she was "safe" and, having thought about what he said, decided that she wanted to be referred to another therapist.

The next day, both Joel and Andy were scheduled to attend the advanced Solution-Focused Brief Therapy training at the Brief Family Therapy Center in Milwaukee, Wisconsin. While there, Joel described the events that had taken place with Mary. This led to a spontaneous role-play with Steve de Shazer taking the part of the therapist. First Joel then Andy acted the part of Mary.

During the course of the role-play, de Shazer persistently asked what it was that first Joel and then Andy (in the role of Mary) wanted to be different. Each time, Joel and Andy went back to describing the problem, only to be met again with the same question, "What do you want to be different?" Finally, the role-played Mary stood up, yelled an expletive, and pretended to walk out. de Shazer's response was to sit quietly and then shrug his shoulders.

On the return flight, Andy and Joel discussed the meaning of the course of events during their role-play with de Shazer. They first noted Steve's insistence on the goal. de Shazer's actions were consistent with his writings (1991): "Without clear, concise ways to know whether it has either failed or succeeded, therapy can go on endlessly . . ." (p. 112).

Miller (1997) wrote about meanings inherent within nonverbal communication. Meaning comes not only from what is said but also from the gestures, guttural utterances, and so forth that occur during the course of a conversation. Meanings that are derived from language result from both the spoken and unspoken. A case in point is the discussion between Andy and Joel about the meaning of de Shazer's shrug. We are not suggesting here what de Shazer may have intended, only what meanings Joel and Andy together made from the gesture. The first was that because the transaction had occurred in the context of the "therapy" session, we could not separate it from the process of the role-play. In the context of therapy, Mary's response (whether in the role-play or in the actual session) could only be (mis)understood as integral to what occurred in the room between Mary and Andy (de Shazer, 1991).

The second derived meaning was that Mary chose to act in the way that she did and this choice was to be respected.[3] Consistent with the assumptions of SFBP, Mary did what she perceived to be in her best interest and made the appropriate choice for her. As therapists, we trust that clients have the abilities and resources to make appropriate decisions for themselves. This stance most likely serves to co-construct competency within the client.

A New Beginning

When Joel and Andy returned to the clinic from Wisconsin, they had a voice message from Mary. She said that she had thought about the previous session further, especially the team's feedback to her, and she had to agree that in the past, therapy had not been particularly helpful to her. She continued that she had decided that it was time to try a different approach and that she wanted to continue working with Andy and the team.

When she returned to see Andy, she clearly stated that her goal was to regain custody of her daughter. Andy asked her what needed to happen, and Mary replied that she had to do several things: (1) she needed to improve her relationship with her daughter so that the visitation supervisor could see and report that progress, (2) she needed to improve her relationship with and demonstrate her ability to follow the advice of the caseworker, and (3) she needed to find ways of expressing her anger and frustration that did not result in hospitalizations because this reinforced her reputation as a "borderline."

During the course of the interview, Andy and Mary worked together to explore the details of the meanings and potential usefulness of each of these elements. Andy was especially careful to include how the various people in Mary's life—her daughter, her foster care caseworker, and the worker supervising her visitations with her daughter—would know that she was making progress. After the midsession break with the team, Andy expressed the team's admiration for Mary's thoughtfulness and decision. The team reiterated that by her actions, Mary was clearly indicating how much she loved her daughter and how serious she was about her goal of regaining custody of the child.

Mary returned the next session and reported the progress that she had noticed. She talked about a very positive visit with her daughter, who seemed to be more affectionate and caring toward Mary. She said that she had made an effort to talk to her supervising worker, who acknowledged how positively the session went. The team expressed their delight in Mary's progress and suggested that she keep noticing what was letting her, the visitation supervisor, and the foster care caseworker know that she continued to make progress.

During the next few sessions, Mary continued to report progress. During one, she told Andy that she would like to invite her caseworker to participate behind the mirror with the team at the next session. Andy and the team wholeheartedly supported the idea. The next session was scheduled for two weeks later and Mary called to confirm that the caseworker would be there.

During Mary's next appointment, the caseworker, sitting behind the mirror, commented on Mary's progress. During the break consultation, the caseworker expressed her amazement at how cooperative Mary had become and how she and Mary had managed to forge a positive working relationship. The caseworker also told the team that the visitation supervisor had likewise commented on how different Mary seemed and how much closer the mother and daughter had become. With the caseworker's permission, the team included her compliments in the feedback to Mary. Mary was delighted and this reinforced for her that her hard work was having a positive effect on everyone.

Mary began the next session by announcing that based upon her progress, she would now be able to see her daughter in unsupervised visits. Mary stated that she was bringing her daughter to the next session so that they could continue to work on their relationship together. True to her word, Mary brought her daughter to the appointment and the team and Andy finally had a chance to meet her and observe the relationship between Mary and the child. The team complimented Mary on how loving she was to her daughter and how they seemed to enjoy each other's company. The team commented that they could not suggest much, except for Mary to keep doing more of what was working.

Mary returned to see Andy and the team a month after the session with her daughter. She discussed the progress that she had made and, when asked to scale her confidence in being able to continue making progress, she rated herself at an 8. She apologetically told Andy that she thought it was time to continue the progress on her own and that she did not need to continue in therapy. She also informed him that she had discussed this with her caseworker, who agreed with the decision. The team expressed its delight that she had decided this and had consulted her caseworker. They agreed that based on her confidence, further sessions were unnecessary, and Mary was assured that if she were to get off track, she could always return.

That was the last time the team and Andy saw Mary. They never discovered whether Mary regained custody of her child. Her reputation in the county seemed to fade, and it appeared that she lost her membership in the mental health Hall of Infamy.

As trainers and teachers in Solution-Focused Brief Therapy, we often are asked with what categories of people SFBP works best. We respond (slightly tongue in cheek) that the approach will work only with individuals who can entertain even the slightest possibility of a better life. As in Mary's case, this was the foundation of a solution-building conversation.

We also are asked whether the approach will work with [*fill in the blank*] diagnosis. This is a difficult question to answer, for we do not work with borderlines, schizophrenics, or agoraphobics; we work with people who seek our help in finding a satisfactory solution to the problem(s) that motivate them to seek help.

NOTES

1. Clients' names and identifying information have been altered.
2. See Chapters 6 and 9 for discussion.
3. To avoid confusion, we are not suggesting that, as therapists, we should allow clients to engage in activities that immediately endanger themselves and others. It generally is recognized that mental health professionals have legal, professional, and probably moral responsibilities to take whatever reasonable actions they are able to in order to address the safety of clients and those who have contact with them. In Mary's case, she had contacted Andy and assured him that she was safe and had made an informed choice.

Chapter 4

"I Have More of a Sound Mind Now"

One of the strengths of the solution-focused brief approach is its inherent adaptability to diverse contexts and populations. Books have been written about SFBP with eating disorders (McFarland, 1995), domestic violence (Lee, Sebold, & Uken, 2003), children and adolescents (Berg & Steiner, 2003), in schools (Metcalf, 1995), parenting (Crawford, 2003), sexual abuse (Dolan, 1991), child protective services (Berg, 2000), and substance misuse (Berg & Miller, 1992), to name a few. In addition, many solution-focused articles are written in numerous professional journals throughout the world. With the publication of this book, this list is now expanded to include use of SFBP with long-term users of the mental health system.

Each application of SFBP has in common with the others the miracle question, scaling questions, exception questions, and questions that project into the future. The application to differing contexts is most likely in the ways in which the various tools are used and/or emphasized. For example, therapy with the client who has been socialized as a mental health patient often is most useful when it is intermittent. As an intensive case manager, Joel had numerous experiences of accompanying his clients to their therapy sessions and listening to the treating clinicians and psychiatrists repeatedly explain to clients the realities of their respective diagnoses and the need to see their therapists weekly as well as to consistently take their medications. We have learned from experience that these clients do not always follow clinicians' prescriptions, and it is thus essential that the clinician tailor therapy to the needs and pace of the client. This may mean having sessions that are not on a set schedule and are fit to the clients' needs rather than tradition.

Clients often comply with suggestions when they are experiencing a crisis or when they are newly discharged from psychiatric hospitals.

Solution-Focused Brief Practice
© 2007 by The Haworth Press, Taylor & Francis Group. All rights reserved.
doi:10.1300/5507_04

However, we recognize that clients have lives outside of mental health clinics and many (if not most) balk at defining themselves as chronic psychiatric patients whose lives seemingly revolve around clinical appointments. Very often, once the crisis has passed, they begin to miss appointments. They then are labeled as "noncompliant" and "resistant" and warned that without adequate treatment they will forever be psychiatric hospital recidivists, which adds more negative expectations upon them. From years of experience, most can predict these conversations, and it becomes one more incentive for avoiding their clinic contacts. In addition, the message that powerful psychiatric medications are lifelong necessities despite their side effects adds another incentive for clients to avoid mental health professionals. Finally, when they are doing well, they do not see the need for attending therapy sessions, which is often contary to prevailing ideas about their treatment. Experienced mental health professionals themselves are well aware that conversations such as those described have had limited success, historically. Yet, many express with exasperation that they do not know what else to do except repeat the admonitions to the clients.

A story exists about a man who was driving past a state psychiatric hospital when he rode over a nail that punctured his tire. He stopped the car, stepped out, and inspected the tire, realizing that he was going to have to use the spare in his trunk. While figuring this out, he noticed a man standing across the street who was having an active conversation with no one in particular. The driver surmised by the appearance and behaviors that the man was a resident of this particular institution.

Hoping to avoid the attention of the psychiatric patient, the man nervously began to change his tire. He opened the trunk and removed the spare, the jack, and the tire tool. He loosened the lug nuts, raised the car, removed the lug nuts, and placed them in the overturned hubcap. The patient now had turned his full attention to the driver, and the driver, realizing this, became even more nervous and accidentally dropped the hubcap. All but three of the lug nuts rolled into a storm drain and were lost. As the man was trying to decide what to do next, the patient slowly strolled across the street, making the driver even more nervous with fantasies of being molested on the spot by some crazy person.

After a few moments, the patient suggested that the driver alternate the spaces so that the lug nuts formed a triangle, which should stabilize the tire and get the driver to the closest auto parts store. Relieved, the driver expressed his perplexity that the patient would be able to come up with such a practical solution. The patient responded, "I may be crazy, but I ain't stupid."

The solution to "noncompliance" requires a set of assumptions about the client and the clinician that are different from the usual; if allowed, and with the help of useful conversations, clients ultimately are responsible and capable of working with therapists to develop goals and treatment plans. Instead of assuming that clients "resist" therapists and treatment, the solution-focused approach assumes that clients give clues about how therapy can work for them and that therapists must cooperate with these clues (de Shazer, 1984). They are more likely to carry through with ideas that they have participated in making, and, when those do not help, are more likely to participate in nonblaming conversations to determine what might be more workable for them. It is clinicians' responsibility to build a collaborative relationship with clients. The team's work with Stephen illustrates these points.

APPRECIATING THE ORDINARY

Stephen was 40 years old. According to his record, he had had a history of psychiatric problems since early childhood. He was first hospitalized at the state psychiatric center at age 17. Since then, he had had multiple hospitalizations in community mental health units as well as the state psychiatric center. The average hospital stays were of relatively long duration, lasting from three to eight weeks. Stephen had had four psychiatric evaluations completed by separate psychiatrists that reflected his history the six years prior to his contact with Joel. Each psychiatrist diagnosed Stephen as schizophrenic: chronic, undifferentiated type. During the course of his years in mental health, Stephen had taken a variety of psychiatric medications, many of which he complained produced side effects.

Stephen had been treated at another community mental health clinic prior to his referral to the clinic where Joel was practicing. Several weeks prior to his referral, the psychiatrist had written, "Patient complains of swollen tongue. Will discontinue [medication]. Moreover, he has been giving variable complaints, verbalizing suicidal ideation then retracting. Now complains of insomnia. I believe he is malingering for attention." This final psychiatric note also stated,

"Stephen, as usual, now requests a return to [medication] several weeks after he requested to have [same medication] changed as ineffective. Things are going round and round with no progress. His family reports that he lies and should not be believed. This, however, leaves open the question of how to track him. . . ."

During the course of the two and one-half years that Joel and the team worked with Stephen, he faithfully attended approximately 20 sessions. After the first, sessions lasted an average of 30 minutes or less. During his prior extensive inpatient and outpatient treatments, Stephen frequently had been labeled noncompliant and resistant. Yet, he presented a very different picture to a solution-focused therapist: cooperative, thoughtful, goal oriented, and motivated. The course of Stephen's work is illustrative of the way in which SFBP is a flexible approach that can be adapted to work with individuals, even those who have had many years of mental health treatment and who have been given labels indicative of serious and persistent mental illness.

When Stephen first met with Joel and the team, he was asked about his goals for therapy.[1] He responded that he would "be getting help with schizophrenia."

J: So, how would you know that you would be getting this help?

S: I would be more outspoken with people.

J: Okay. How will those people who know you—your father, your mother, your sister—see you being more outspoken?

S: I'll tell them how I feel and when I'm upset.

J: Right, and how will that be helpful?

S: Then they can help me, make me feel better.

J: What do they do that's helpful when you let them know how you feel?

S: They talk to me, they give me suggestions of what I can do and I try them.

J: Really? And that works?

S: Yeah, it works fine.

In this initial interchange, Stephen's goal was clarified. Notice how Joel stayed with Stephen's words and built each question on the previous answer. As is often the case, we find that exceptions to the problems occur naturally and become apparent as the conversation progresses. Stephen began by explaining what he wanted to be different. After a few exchanges, Joel shifted to a very different question. Rather than using the future or subjunctive, he asked Stephen an exception question: what his family already was doing that was helpful. This served two major functions: (1) it began the process of assessing the community supports that Stephen could use to help him achieve his goals, and (2) it shifted the conversation to Stephen's life between therapy sessions.

Community Supports

We often forget that psychotherapy is a relatively recent discipline that has enjoyed cautious acceptance for only the past 30 years or less. People have not always sought a therapist when they experienced difficult times. In the past, people utilized their social resources: their communities, families, or friends, or their churches, mosques, or synagogues. In SFBP, we help people to reconnect with those resources. If therapists become the clients' major social and emotional support, they become divorced from the very resources in their life situations that will maintain, encourage, and support them in the future and for the long term. Therapists are more helpful when they help clients realize and utilize the resources that already exist in their environments. This is why Joel asked Stephen what his family already did that helped him.

Joel recalls that he once was on a team behind the mirror with another client. The therapist had asked the client a similar question about her community resources and she insisted that she lived alone, was isolated, and had no family or friends in the area. The therapist, realizing that pursuing the client's social resources further would likely not be fruitful and might possibly be off-putting for the client, went on to explore other topics. When the client returned several weeks later, she excitedly related to the therapist how the day after her last session, she happened to meet a neighbor in the hall of their apartment building. The client continued, saying that she and the neighbor had exchanged greetings and talked briefly and that she had invited the neighbor in for a cup of coffee. As the client and neighbor spent some time together, chatting over a cup of coffee, both became surprised how much they had in common and agreed that they wanted to continue their coffee breaks together. The client expressed amazement that she would do such a thing as approach this neighbor—an act that she described as out of character. She also expressed pleasure at the results of her newly realized assertiveness.

Between-Sessions Focus

Let us assume for a moment that most people average 16 waking hours each day in which to live their lives. Let us further suppose that a weekly therapy session lasts 50 minutes, the standard practice in most community mental health clinics. This suggests that most clients live in the world outside of therapy for at least 111 waking hours each week. How many experiences might a client potentially have in those 111 hours? In how many conversations might a client participate within those 111 hours? How many of those experiences and conversations might affect clients' thinking, behaviors, and/or feelings in very profound and life-changing ways?

Because change is always happening, we believe that changes that happen between sessions are important. When the focus of therapy is restricted solely to the clients' experiences in consultation offices, therapists lose the possibilities inherent in the myriad encounters and in the potential to make useful meaning of each one. Lambert (1992) suggested that experiences during the time outside of therapy account for 40 percent of changes that happen during a course of therapy. It is wise for therapists to take advantage of these experiences.

I'd Be More Normal

J: So, Stephen, I have a strange question I want to ask you. I ask it because it will be helpful to me to know what you want to be different in your life. Okay?

S: Sure.

J: Let's suppose that after we talk today, you're going to leave here and do what you normally do [Stephen nods]. Tonight, you're going to go to sleep, and let's suppose that while you're sleeping, some miracle happens. The miracle is that the problems that brought you here to see me disappear, just like that [therapist snaps his fingers]. But you can't know about this miracle yet because it happened while you were sleeping. The only way you

can know about the miracle is what happens differently tomorrow. That's my question, what will be different tomorrow after
the miracle?

S: I wouldn't have to go into a [psychiatric] hospital ever again. I'd be
more normal.

J: Wow, what would be happening instead?

S: Maybe I'd have a job or something.

J: What kind of job?

S: I used to work in a workshop, but they made me leave because I got
into trouble. Maybe I could go back there.

J: What would be different?

S: I'd do my job and not bother anyone—they said I harassed a
woman there.

J: Okay, so what else would be different?

S: I'd take my medication like I'm supposed to. I usually do, though.

J: How's that helpful to you?

S: It helps me keep my thoughts straight and I don't hear things as
much as I used to.

J: What else do you do that's helpful to you?

S: I take long walks, I pray, I talk to my friends. I talk to my mother,
my father, and my sister.

Joel began asking the miracle question by first creating a logical
context. He stated that it would be a way of making greater sense of
Stephen's goal and that Stephen's answers would be helpful in the
therapy. While asking the question, Joel carefully watched Stephen's
reactions to ensure Stephen's comprehension.

Stephen responded with a negative outcome: "I wouldn't go into a
hospital again." Joel's response was to move from what was not going
to be happening to what was going to happen instead. Few possibilities exist in an absence of behavior. The potential that the client will
leave the session with a sense of direction increases as the therapist
converts the descriptions of the lack of problems to descriptions of
alternative, solution behaviors.

Joel then asked Stephen for greater detail about what he meant by
having a job. Joel's assumption was that the more the therapist helps
to fill in details of a solution picture, the more real the solutions be-

come. This in turn increases the probability of something useful happening between sessions.

Two of Stephen's responses invited the therapist into a problem-focused conversation. In each case, Joel remained focused on questions that enlarged on Stephen's vision of positive change. In a very practical way, these interactions illustrate the difference between solution-building versus problem-solving conversations.

I Wouldn't Need to Ever Go to a Hospital Again

J: Stephen, let's say that I have a scale from zero to ten. Ten on the scale is the miracle we just talked about; zero is the farthest from that you can imagine. Where would you put things today?

S: I'd say a four.

J: A four, wow! What makes you say four?

S: Well, I still need therapy.

J: Of course. How is four different from zero?

S: Well, my family helps me, reading the Bible keeps me calm, and I take my medicine. That helps.

Scaling is a particularly useful tool for promoting exception conversations. Logically, any number on the scale above 0 indicates that exceptions to the problem do exist (Berg & de Shazer, 1993). Even when clients respond that they are at 0, we usually find it helpful to ask about a recent time when they would estimate that their situation was higher than 0. Most recall a time when no exceptions to the problem existed. The therapist then asks where the client put himself or herself on the scale at that time. If a client insists that they have never had a time when they were above 0, the therapist might wonder aloud whether the goal is realistic. Clearly, it is our perspective that the client—not the therapist—is responsible for constructing and achieving a realistic goal. However, the therapist may need to help clients identify realistic goals. de Shazer (personal communication, November 5, 2004) pointed out that problems can be solved; some things are situations and cannot (e.g., a physical disability). SFBP focuses on problems that can be solved, or it reframes situations in some way. For example, the therapist might ask a client with goals of winning the lottery what difference winning the lottery would make for them. This difference might then become the goal.

When the miracle question has been asked, we find that it is simpler to set 10 as the miracle. In our experience, it is common for clients initially to give a problem-focused response to scaling, explaining why they are not at 10. Stephen's response is very typical of this. Joel simply normalized the response ("of course") and followed up with a solution-building question ("how is four different from zero"). Interestingly, we often find that once the therapist reverses the meaning of the scale (why not 0 versus why not 10), clients respond similarly to subsequent scales.

J: Right! How do those things help you?
S: They help a lot. My mom and dad give me good suggestions.
J: Like what?
S: Stay calm, take my medicine, and don't be alone too much.

A major result of solution-focused conversations is that they develop richly detailed solution pictures. As we suggest in Chapter 9, language co-constructs reality. A corollary of this concept is that the greater the detail, the more real and abundant the possibilities become. That is, the more we can clearly describe details of a future, the more likely we are to be able to make that future happen and to envision even more possible futures. In this dialogue, it is not enough that Stephen named the changes, but that together Joel and Stephen expanded on the details of exceptions. This increased the probability that Stephen would continue to do more of what had been working for him and to notice more solutions. In the context of SFBP, when a therapist seeks small details of the solution picture, the results tend to be expansive.

J: Sounds like good advice. So, how would you know that five is happening?
S: I wouldn't need to ever go to a hospital again.
J: That sounds a bit large.
S [Laughs] I guess that's more like ten. I think I would take my medicine when I'm supposed to.
J: How would that be helpful?
S: It keeps me calm and I don't hear voices—at least not too much.

The initial scaling served to create a context for a conversation about exceptions (how is 4 different from 0). The next set of questions expanded on future possibilities.

When clients respond to the question of what would be different at one number higher on the scale, our instinct is to make sure that the client's response is realistic. Joel suggested that Stephen's answer may be higher than 5 on the scale. Stephen confirmed that staying out of the hospital is much higher, and he continued with a more realistic expectation: "I would take my medicine when I'm supposed to."

J: Yeah. I have another one of these crazy scales, is that okay?

S: Sure.

J: If ten on the same scale was that all the good things you're doing are because of you and zero is it's all the medicine, where would you put yourself on that scale?

S: I'd say five.

J: Great! Why five?

S: I take my medicine on time, and I do things that calm me down.

J: Like the things you mentioned before: read your Bible, take walks, and take the advice of your family?

S: Yeah.

Clients who have been in the mental health system for many years often attribute positive changes to their medications. Although we will expand on our orientation toward psychiatric medications in a later chapter, as SFB practitioners we see our responsibility as one of co-constructing useful conversations about psychiatric medications. One way of co-constructing that conversation is to focus on the client's agency in the change process.

With Stephen, Joel did this simply by setting a scale where one pole represented the client as the agent of change and the other pole, the medication. Stephen's response is very typical: he placed himself somewhere in the middle. Joel's follow-up question elicited Stephen's response about what he does that moves him toward his goal. To use his agency, Joel emphasized what Stephen does in addition to taking medicine. In another conversation, an SFBP therapist might ask the client how she or he helps the medicine to work, also increasing self-efficacy.

Course of Treatment

What is probably most notable about Joel's and the team's work with Stephen is how ordinary the process became. Yet, given Stephen's previous treatment history and labels as noncompliant and resistant, the ordinariness is what makes this case so extraordinary.

John Shotter (1994) reflected on this phenomenon:

> But it is how people re-collect their past due to their need to act "into" an interest in the future, thus to "reshape" what has been—not how they must act out of a fixed past—that is crucial, not just in personal psychotherapy, but in us curing what Wittgenstein saw as a sickness of our time. Where, as he saw it, an aspect of that sickness lies in our incapacity to wonder, our incapacity to recognize that the strange, the unique, the novel, the unknown, and the extraordinary lie hidden within our everyday mundane activity. (p. 71)

Gale Miller (personal communication, October, 1997) stated that when he observed Insoo Kim Berg working with a client, he noticed that she often responded with "Wow" to a client at times when she could just as well have responded, "So what." Miller described how solution-focused practitioners have the capacity to appreciate the extraordinary acts that people do in the course of their ordinary lives.

The ability to find the extraordinary within the ordinary is essential to working with long-term users of mental health services. The ability of therapists and clients to structure conversations about differences is crucial to instilling a sense of hope and expectation for both. Without a hopeful perspective, therapists experience frustration and hopelessness that accompanies the perception that nothing changes; the work with clients then is for naught. The perception of hope and expectation and the ability of the therapist to build on even the smallest differences engender a sense of excitement and curiosity for working with clients.

I Have More of a Sound Mind Now

Following is a verbatim of a typical session with Stephen using an observing team.

J: So, it's been three weeks?

S: Yeah, three weeks.

J: Okay, so, what's been better?

S: I'm going to River Club [a local psychosocial program]. That's a good thing. Yesterday we went to Southern County—a conference. We went to talk about what our program is all about. I went with four other people.

J: So, were you on a panel or something?

S: Yeah, we talked about what we feel is good about the program.

J: So you were part of this conference—wow. How did they choose you?

S: They chose five people.

J: How did you get chosen?

S: I said, "can I go?" and they said I was welcome to go.

J: What happened there that was helpful?

S: We gave feedback. I told them who I was and where I was from.

J: That's great. What else are you doing?

S: I've been going to the church. I have friends there. The minister has been counseling me on religious things.

J: Good. How has that been helpful?

S: That's been helpful. I feel at home at that church. It's like a family there. It's warm. There are a lot of friendly people there. I've been helping out at River Club with the donations.

J: You're still going there?

S: I love it. Before, I didn't want to go. I tried it before but I didn't like it. Now I like it much better.

J: What do you think is different about you that makes the difference in your liking it?

S: Giving things more of chance to work before making the decision.

J: What told you that that would be helpful to you?

S: My mom gave me feedback. She told me I should go and try it.

J: How did you stay so open—how did you not make a decision before you tried it?

S: Being patient and giving things a chance.

J: When did you first start noticing you were thinking that way?

S: Back in September when I first started going.

J: So, on a scale where ten is you're on track, where would you put things?

S: Ten.

J: Confidence that you can stay on track—where would you put yourself there?

S: I'm not too confident but kind of confident.

J: Where?

S: I'll say eight.

J: Eight. What gives you that confidence?

S: My faith in God.

J: Okay, faith in God. What else?

S: My friends, support from my family. Things like that.

J: What are you doing that gives you confidence?

S: Going to my programs, being responsible. Keeping my appointments.

J: Anything else before I take the break?

[Stephen stated that he reported to his psychiatrist that he was hearing chainlike sounds. The psychiatrist suggested that he discuss this with his therapist. This portion will be presented in the section on turning problems into solutions.]

S: Also, I've had an older woman as a friend for about four years and she turned against me. She told me not to call her in the morning, so I called her at four in the afternoon. She told me that she didn't want me to call her any more.

J: Wow, so how did you deal with that?

S: Well, I expected it when she told me not to call her in the morning because she's busy. I knew it was an excuse. I thought to myself that I had other friends and my church and my family and that if she didn't want to be friends with me anymore, I wouldn't call her anymore.

J: So, I'm going to take a break and meet with the team back there.

[Joel returns with feedback from the team.]

J: The thing we're the most impressed about is how thoughtful you are about yourself. We're also impressed with how focused you are on what works. You're figuring out things for yourself. It seems like you have a lot of people who support you and give you advice.

But you're the one who makes it happen. Advice is easy; taking it is hard work. Another example of figuring things out is how you've learned to give things a chance. One of the team members said how impressed they were that you spoke at this conference. You're reaching out to the community and spending less time at home. The church has been like a home to you; it's warm and you made friends there. There's River Club—you have friends there. These are signs to us that you are becoming more and more normal. You said that was one of your goals—to be more normal.

S: I'd say I have more of a sound mind now.

J: Yes. More of a sound mind, exactly. We're really impressed how you handled things when this woman turned against you. Of course it hurt, but you handled it. You said in your mind, "I have other friends." You have the church, you have River Club, and you have other friends. You didn't dwell on her turning against you. You focused on what your alternatives are. That's impressive; that's hard work.

S: I've come a long way; I don't want to go back into the hospital. That's why I handled it that way.

J: Yes, it's been almost a year.

S: Next month will be one year.

J: The other thing that tells us that you are thinking in a more normal way: the way you treat this thing called schizophrenia. You've not allowed that to be your focus. It's something that you handle but it's not you—it's just a part of you. Our sense is you're thinking more and more that way about yourself. Our suggestion is that you keep doing what works for you in your life and keep learning about what does work.

Life Happens

The real successes of therapy become evident in the way individuals handle issues that occur naturally in the course of their lives, not just responses to questions in therapy sessions. Most people turn to their social resources to deal with life's vagaries. For example, most of us accept sadness as a normal response when a loved one dies. The emotions can momentarily be overwhelming and even debilitating. We turn to our friends and families; we seek out the comfort of our social and religious institutions to help us through difficult times.

Sometimes, we might seek out a therapist briefly to help us put our situation in a more useful perspective. With time and support, we most often figure out how to get ourselves back on track and to go on with our lives.

Those who have been conditioned by years of therapy in mental health settings often utilize psychiatric hospitalization as their major resource for support. Hospitals are useful and practical places that can help protect people who are at risk for hurting themselves or others while they regain a sense of stability. The downsides of psychiatric hospitalizations are the tendency within the medical model to reify diagnoses (de Shazer, 1998), reduce people to their labels, and isolate individuals from their community supports.

In the midst of Stephen's sessions with Joel and the team, his father died. Naturally feeling sad about the death of someone who had supported him and had a profound influence on his life, Stephen talked about being "depressed" and went to an inpatient mental health unit for an evaluation. He was admitted, spent a day and a half as an inpatient and, realizing that he no longer needed to be hospitalized, requested discharge. The staff agreed that Stephen no longer needed to be hospitalized and he was discharged from the hospital less than two days after admission. This was the only time in the two and a half years that Joel and the team worked with Stephen that he had been hospitalized, a considerable reduction in the use of the hospital as a resource for him.

In the spring of 1998, Stephen contacted Joel by phone. He told Joel that his mother, with whom he lived, had died and that he was feeling very sad. Joel's response was to normalize the sadness simply by stating, "Of course, who wouldn't be?" Joel went on to ask Stephen what was helping him get through this rough period. Stephen replied that his family surrounded him and the members of his church also were providing much needed support. Joel then asked Stephen to scale, in which 10 was that he was naturally going through a tough time but that he was confident that he would be able to get through it with the support of his family and friends, and 0 meant that he would be going to the hospital as soon as he hung up the phone. Stephen replied that he experienced himself at a 10, and they discussed what made him so confident. Stephen was not hospitalized, and, based on his vastly improved functioning, his sister agreed that Stephen should live with her and her family.

It's Not a Problem; It's a Solution

Clients often experience symptoms that are reflective of biological processes gone awry. Auditory and visual hallucinations are common examples. When clients report that they hear voices or see things that no one else sees or hears, we follow the basic precepts of SFBP: begin with the client's reality, the meaning they make of that reality, and the differences they would identify as reasonable goals for change. We see our jobs as solution-focused therapists as helping to create useful meanings with clients about the events that happen in their lives. Certainly, newer medications have proven useful in controlling psychiatric symptoms with fewer side effects. SFBP tools are the conversations that we have with clients and how those conversations serve to co-construct useful realities that help them function as well as they possibly can.

Milton Erickson stated that he had no particular governing theory, and when working with clients, he simply observed and utilized whatever the clients brought—experiences, thoughts, feelings, behaviors, symptoms, etc.—that would help develop solutions (Rosen, 1991). As solution-focused practitioners, our interest is to have conversations that go beyond the details of problems and instead build on the details of solutions. We ask ourselves, "What will clients take from the conversations that will prove helpful to them?"

Stephen reported to the psychiatrist that he was experiencing auditory hallucinations. In turn, the psychiatrist directed Stephen to discuss this with his therapist. Stephen explained to Joel that at times he heard what sounded like chains rattling. We have trained ourselves to listen with "solution-building ears." The phrase "at times" implies the sounds were not constant, so Joel asked Stephen about times that he either did not hear the chains or heard them less. Stephen responded that he did not hear the chains while at River Club.

J: So, when you're at River Club, you don't hear it.

S: When I'm here, I don't hear it either.

J: What's different at River Club? What's different here?

S: I also don't hear it in church.

J: So what's different here, at River Club, and at church?

S: At River Club, there's noise that blocks it out—same thing in church. When I'm alone, I hear it. It's scary. I asked my mom whether she hears it. She told me it's probably in my mind.

J: What told you to ask your mom? That's impressive! You did an experiment—you did some research.

S: [Laughs] Yeah, I asked my mom.

J: How did you figure out how to do that?

S: I wanted to make sure it wasn't something going on in the whole family. My sister said she didn't hear it; my mom said she didn't hear it.

J: Once you found out it wasn't real, how did that change things for you?

S: It's still kind of scary. I know it's not real.

J: That's helpful?

S: It helps relieve some of the scariness.

J: What are other times at your house when you don't you hear it?

S: I don't hear it during the day, only at night.

J: What's different during the day?

S: During the day I'm busy. My mind is on other things.

J: So, when you're busy, your mind is on other things.

S: Only when I'm by myself and alone, I hear it. (Berg and Dolan, 2001, pp. 165 & 166)

The conversation built on Stephen's simple statement that he heard the chains "at times." As practitioners develop the ability to listen with solution-building ears, we begin to appreciate the potential for building on ever smaller exceptions. We consistently listen for ways to invite clients into solution-focused conversations because we know from experience that solution-talk increases the potential for continued solution-talk. Joel's and Stephen's conversation is a good example of the practical way that solution-focused conversations build on exceptions.

Joel began this conversation with one exception: when Stephen was at River Club, he did not hear the chains. Very quickly, Stephen spontaneously recalled a second exception. Joel asked what the two exceptions had in common. Stephen raised a third exception, and Joel inquired as to how all three exceptions were similar. Stephen provided a very plausible explanation: a noise blocks it out. Stephen then expanded the explanation and concluded that when his "mind is on other things" he is not bothered by the sound of chains.

When we converse within a problem-focused language game, problems can be viewed as both constant and unyielding. However, it is clear that when conversation focuses on exceptions to problems, constancy dissolves. In fact, Stephen told us very early that the problem existed only when he was alone.

In this conversation Stephen informed Joel that he had asked his mother and sister whether they were hearing sounds of chains. More traditional therapy approaches would recognize this as an example of "reality testing." Joel credited Stephen with coming up with this idea on his own. Joel then asked Stephen what this meant for him, and in so doing, built on and reinforced how useful it was for Stephen to use his community resources.

J: If I had a scale where ten is it only happens at night, it's really not scary, and you can ignore it and zero is the opposite, where would you put yourself right now?

S: I'd say five. I control it a little bit, not much.

J: How do you control it?

S: Take my medicine on time. Eat right—I'm diabetic. That has something to do with it.

J: How does the medicine help?

S: Which one? For diabetes or my schizophrenia?

J: Either one.

S: It stabilizes me, keeps me calm, and I sleep well.

J: And controlling your diet, how is that helpful?

S: If I eat well . . . If I drink coffee, I hear it more. So I cut down on coffee.

J: What else gets you to five?

S: I pray a lot, that helps. I talk to people. When I get angry, I hear it even more.

J: So, how do you keep from getting angry?

S: Go to River Club and talk to people there.

J: Since you've been doing that and getting less angry, what have you noticed is different?

S: I haven't been hearing it as much.

J: What else do you do to get to that five?

S: Look at my [car] models; sometimes I draw. I go to the library.

J: How are those things helpful?

S: They help pretty good.

J: How would you know that six is happening?

S: Keeping more active and controlling it more.

J: What about at night, how would you know six is happening then?

S: Probably keeping busier—finding something to do to keep busy.

J: What could you do that would be helpful?

S: Call a friend I could trust.

J: What else?

S: Exercise, do sit-ups. Read the Bible or books.

J: So, on a confidence scale where ten is you're really sure that these things will help and zero is the opposite, where are you?

S: Ten. The other thing is going to bed later.

J: You have lots of good ideas. How did you come up with them?

S: That was what my dad said to do.

J: What other ideas did Dad have that are helpful to you?

S: He said, "don't think too much. Don't sit around and daydream. Stay busy." (Berg and Dolan, 2001, pp. 166 & 167)

The previous interactive sequence is a good example of the usefulness of scaling questions. Numbers by their very nature invite concrete pictures. Solution-focused therapists realize that scaling numbers have no meaning except for the meanings that we attribute to them through our conversations with clients. Berg and de Shazer (1993) addressed this concept:

> Scales allow both therapist and client to use the way language works naturally by agreeing upon terms (i.e., numbers) and a concept (a scale where ten stands for the goal and zero stands for an absence of progress toward the goal) that is obviously multiple and flexible. Since neither therapist nor client can be absolutely certain what the other means by the use of a particular word or concept, scaling questions allow them to jointly construct a way of talking about things that are hard to describe, including progress toward the client's goal(s). (p. 19)

Joel initially set what could be viewed as a "scariness" scale. Stephen then changed the meaning of the scale and addressed control as the issue. Joel quickly accepted Stephen's meaning and asked how Stephen controlled the sounds to the extent that he did. Stephen set the scale at 5. If we accept Stephen's meaning of the scale, 5 has two possible overall meanings, each one equally valid: 5 is higher than 0 through 4, 5 is lower than 6 through 10. Our experience is that the former more functionally serves a solution-building conversation than the latter.

In fact, building a conversation around how 5 indicates progress yields a wealth of strategies that Stephen had developed on his own to minimize the effect of the sounds: medication, diet, talking to people at River Club, looking at his car models, drawing, and going to the library. When Joel simply asked, "What else?" Stephen added going to bed early, exercising, reading, and following the advice of his father: "Don't think too much. Don't sit around and daydream. Stay busy."

Joel reinforced the solution-building process by asking Stephen to scale his confidence that the ideas would be helpful. Stephen's response that he perceived himself as 10 on the scale suggested to Joel that Stephen would very likely leave the conversation with confidence that he had developed useful and practical solutions that he could employ because they had worked in the past. Moreover, the conversation served to deconstruct the idea that the problem is constant and out of Stephen's control.[2] What is particularly impressive is that all of this took place within a thirty-minute session.

CONVERSATIONS THAT MAKE
A DIFFERENCE: NADINE

Nadine was a 16-year-old high school junior referred to an intensive day treatment (IDT) program where Joel was working as a clinician. IDT was structured as a short-term (approximately 30-day) program for adolescents who were experiencing a mental health crisis or who were being returned to the community after psychiatric hospitalization. IDT combined both clinical and educational services with the goal of stabilizing the adolescent and gradually transitioning him or her back to the home school district.

Nadine's home district referred her to IDT after discharge from a private psychiatric hospital. According to her record, she had complained of hearing voices, especially someone that she identified as Lucy. Nadine characterized Lucy as being angry with her, and she expressed concern that Lucy would impel her to harm herself. On the particular day of this reported conversation with Joel, Nadine had had difficulty concentrating on her work and complained that Lucy was especially intrusive. In the past, similar events frequently heralded psychiatric hospitalizations. The IDT classroom teacher had suggested to Nadine that she sit in the clinical office so she could "calm down" before returning to the classroom. Nadine's usual therapist was not at IDT that day. Joel had had previous contact with Nadine in group therapy. He approached Nadine and asked if it would be all right with her if they talked together. She agreed.

J: Well, thanks for agreeing to talk with me. I'm very curious about something and have a strange question for you, okay?

N: Yes.

J: How is Lucy helpful to you?

N: She wants me to be happy.

J: Right. And how does she know when you are happy?

N: I smile, I laugh, I talk to my parents and my friends and I can concentrate on my schoolwork.

J: So, when you smile, laugh, talk to your parents, and concentrate on your schoolwork, what does Lucy do?

N: She goes away. She wants to go away; she doesn't want to be with me.

J: And is that all right with you if she goes away.

N: Yes.

J: Great! What will tell her that it's okay to go away?

N: When I stay happy and can do my schoolwork.

Although it is true for most people, a sense of respect is especially crucial when working with adolescents. Joel begins by making sure that Nadine is willing to engage in the conversation. From Joel's perspective, it was not enough to remove Nadine from the classroom. Meanings (whether useful or not) are created within a social context (de Shazer, 1991), and it is our experience that social isolation does not provide an opportunity for deconstruction of problems or the construction of workable solutions.

In the past, Nadine's talk about Lucy served to excite the system around her. Her parents, teachers, and friends became anxious and fearful. They viewed the presence of Lucy as a sign that Nadine was out of control and therefore required hospitalization. Once hospitalized, she fell behind in her work, which served to increase her fear and sense of being out of control, which in turn exacerbated the psychiatric behaviors. Of course, this served to make her social system more anxious, and it is easy to see the feedback loop that existed.

Joel took a very different tack: He asked Nadine how Lucy was helpful. Dr. Sidney Rosen (1991) wrote about a woman who had seen Milton Erickson, complaining that she was disturbed by hallucinations of naked men. According to Rosen, Erickson suggested that she leave her naked men in his closet and periodically return to ensure that they were still there. Because Erickson had treated the hallucinations as real objects, they could be locked in a closet or shipped in an envelope. In other words, they could be manipulated (Rosen, 1991).

Similarly, Joel accepted Nadine's reality, and rather than avoid the topic of Lucy, he co-constructed with Nadine ways in which Lucy was helpful to her and the conditions in which Lucy would be able to leave. It is important to note that Lucy's leaving was not Joel's agenda. Had Nadine not raised this possibility, the conversation would have continued in a different (and hopefully as helpful) direction. In fact, Joel asked Nadine if it was her desire for Lucy to go away. As solution-focused practitioners, we do not enter the conversation with preconceived goals except to simply invite the client into a solution-building conversation, as well as inviting them to maintain this conversation. It is up to the client to determine the goal.

J: Hmmm, to help me understand better, is it okay if I ask you one of those crazy scales? [Nadine had been asked scaling questions because Joel frequently used them with the adolescents in group therapy.]

N: [Laughs] Sure.

J: On a scale of zero to ten, where ten is that Lucy thinks it's all right for her to leave you forever, where would you put things today?

N: Three.

J: Three. Wow, how come up to three?

N: A lot of times, I'm happy and can concentrate. That makes her happy and she goes away.

J: What is it that helps you be happy and concentrate?

N: I talk to my friends; they help a lot just talking to me. My parents help me, too.

J: Right, so what do your friends do that helps you be happy?

N: Nothing special. We just hang out together, maybe go to the mall or a movie.

J: And that's helpful to you?

N: Yeah, I enjoy being with them. That takes my mind off my problems.

J: What do your parents do that helps you?

N: They encourage me, they tell me how smart I am, they keep me busy. Sometimes, my father acts silly and he makes me laugh.

J: Let's suppose that things went to four on that scale. What would you notice different?

N: I'd be able to concentrate better on my schoolwork.

J: So, that's important to you?

N: Yes, I want to go to college.

J: Great. When are there times that you are able to concentrate better?

N: I'm finding it easier now, but it's still hard.

J: Sure. What part of it is easier?

N: Well, it helps here at IDT because there are not so many people in the classroom and [the classroom teacher] helps me with my work. I'm able to catch up on a lot of the work I missed.

J: What you say certainly makes a lot of sense to me. Especially that Lucy wants you to be happy and although she wants to go away, she thinks you might still need her.

N: She wants to leave and she wants me to be happy.

J: Right. I'm wondering: do you think that you might be ready to go back to the classroom now?

N: I think so; I'm much calmer than before.

J: That's good. I'll walk you back. Thanks for taking the time to talk with me. It was very helpful.

N: Sure.

Nadine had suggested a useful scale: 10 is when Lucy is ready to leave permanently. As Nadine and Joel made meaning of the 3 on the scale, the exceptions began to emerge, as did her resources. Very often, when a system begins to focus exclusively on a client's psychiatric issues, the healthy and normal part of the individual that exists at the same time is lost. It is seductive to enter into an either/or way of thinking about clients: either they are sick or they are healthy; either they are abnormal or they are normal. SFBP recognizes the both/and nature of humanity.

The conversation with Nadine demonstrates how therapists and clients can have conversations that emphasize the healthy parts of an individual. Nadine is not only the young woman with a psychiatric history; at the same time, she likes to "hang out" with her friends, laugh with her silly father, has the goal of attending college, and wants to be successful in school.

A DIFFERENCE THAT MAKES A DIFFERENCE

Both Stephen's and Nadine's cases illustrate how the assumptions that practitioners make can result in very different conversations and how different conversations have the ability to co-construct very different realities. Joel assumed that Stephen and Nadine were competent, were capable of figuring out what was likely to work, were not defined by their diagnoses or their problems, and therefore were multidimensional people with internal (personal) and external (social) resources.

The assumptions of SFBP drove a conversational set that created a very different experience and reality for both Stephen and Nadine from that which they had experienced with other mental health professionals. At no time did Joel express to either Stephen or Nadine that their respective diagnoses defined them as psychically fragile or brittle, or that it was predictive of any future course of their lives. At the same time, he did not argue about the diagnoses; he accepted the labels as realities (as words) but not the limitations that often are assumed to accompany them. Whether the labels "really" suggested illness was never a topic of conversation.

During his time with Stephen, Joel never admonished Stephen that he needed to take his medication or see a therapist. Yet, during the course of the two and a half years, Stephen was consistent about using medication and therapy. Joel questioned Stephen several times as to whether continued sessions were useful to him. In each case, Stephen decided that he wished to continue the sessions and that the contacts with Joel and the team helped him stay on track. Joel and his team never assumed that they knew what was most useful to Stephen, and therefore relied on Stephen to decide whether and when to return.

The sessions themselves focused on what Stephen was doing in his life that was helping him achieve his goal. The sessions averaged 30 minutes in length, including the time to consult with the team and return with compliments. When difficulties did arise, they were normalized as expected parts of a process toward achieving Stephen's goal.

The conversations with Stephen focused on useful information he had learned from the episodes, how the information would be useful for him in the future, how he managed to keep the situations from getting worse, and, ultimately, what would be useful in getting him back on track.

While Stephen was seen over a period of two and a half years, the actual number of sessions was about 20. In his introduction to Yvonne Dolan's (1991) book, de Shazer stated that brief therapy ". . . simply means therapy that takes as few sessions as possible, not even one more than is necessary, for you to develop a satisfactory solution" (p. *x*).

The single conversation with Nadine lasted no more than 20 minutes. Yet, the richness of the conversation and the wide scope it covered within that brief period is quite evident. Some were concerned that day that Nadine would require another hospitalization. In fact, she returned to her classroom and was able to concentrate and complete her schoolwork; she was not hospitalized.

Nadine successfully returned to her home school district not long after the conversation with Joel. She sent a letter to IDT several weeks later, stating that she was doing well, and thanking the staff for their help. She specifically mentioned the conversation with Joel as having a positive impact on her.

CONCLUSION

Joel left the agency shortly after Stephen decided that he no longer needed to continue in therapy. In his last contact with the clinic staff, Joel learned that with the exception of the brief hospitalization after his father died, Stephen had not been admitted to a psychiatric hospital in over five years, that he continued to live with his sister's family, that he attended church regularly, and that he still was active in River Club. Both Stephen and Nadine demonstrate that a simple conversation or series of conversations that take clients' goals literally, and remain focused on clients' personal and social resources, can have a profound and lasting effect.

NOTES

1. Portions of this interview first appeared in Berg and Dolan (2001).
2. The next chapter will further address deconstruction as a solution-building tool.

Chapter 5

"Agoraphobia" and "Me"
Are Not Synonymous

Therapists and clients say many things during the normal course of a therapy session. As therapists, we often do not know what we'll say that will have a profound impact on clients (and we cannot predict what clients will say that will have a profound impact on us). We frequently are taken aback when clients return and state how meaningful to them something was that we said in a previous session—very often something that we took as insignificant or do not even recall saying.

Clients come to us with a set of beliefs, misunderstandings, and alleged truisms that frequently are part of language games that maintain their views of themselves as dysfunctional, limited, and disabled. As solution-focused therapists, we attempt to have conversations that challenge these long-held beliefs and thereby expand opportunities for clients to see realistic, positive possibilities. Our hope is that these different language games develop and maintain clients' views of themselves as functional, capable, and competent.

DE- AND RE-CONSTRUCTION

de Shazer (1988) explained the notion of deconstructing the frame:

> Developing some doubt about the global frames involves a process that can best be called deconstructing the frame. During the interview, first as the therapist helps the client search for exceptions, and then as the therapist helps the client imagine a future without the complaint, the therapist is implicitly breaking down the frame into smaller and smaller pieces. As it becomes clearer

Solution-Focused Brief Practice
© 2007 by The Haworth Press, Taylor & Francis Group. All rights reserved.
doi:10.1300/5507_05

and clearer that a global frame is involved, the therapist helps the client break it down further into its component parts. The purpose of breaking the frame down is threefold:

1. the therapist is showing his [sic] acceptance of the client just as he is by listening closely and carefully asking questions,
2. the therapist is attempting to introduce some doubt about the global frame, and
3. the therapist is searching for a piece of the frame's construction upon which a solution can be built. (p. 102)

Campbell, Elder, Gallagher, Simon, and Taylor (1999) defined the restructuring process:

Many clients define the problem in ways that limit solutions, such as chemical imbalance, abusive partners, misbehaving children, or a diagnostic label. Solution-focused therapy uses questions to create awareness of options. Restructuring statements are effective tools in this process. We have found recurring themes that can be presented to the client as more useful ways of thinking about the problem. (p. 28)

Restructuring is not an attempt to find the underlying structures that support either troubles or solutions. Rather, it is a process that reconstructs a frame around problems so that it is more possible for solutions to be built. The frame is reconstructed from "problem with no solution" to "problem plus solutions."

Following is the story of David and the conversations that challenged him to think differently.

David was 43 years old and lived with his elderly mother. Although he graduated from a prestigious university, he had had minimal employment. At the time of the first contact with the therapist (Joel) and the team, David had most recently worked for about a year as a security guard at a food distribution center.

David said that he had experienced "panic attacks" in the past. He attributed this to having been bullied with no protection from his teachers and principal during his junior high school career. According to David, this left him with the inability to work and a seething anger that he stated usually was directed toward his mother. He explained that he is "short" with her and that he sometimes broke dishes when the rage became especially intolerable. He denied that he had at anytime been physically abusive to her.

David had been in therapy at another clinic for seven years, and involved in therapy for many years before that. He described the therapy progress as limited, but understood this not as deficiencies in the therapy but the tenacity of his "agoraphobia." The situation came to a head when he sent a facsimile to his junior high school, attributing his current mental health problems to their lack of concern and ineptitude. According to David, he suggested that the school should be burned down as rightful retribution. The school officials became concerned and contacted the police. David was arrested and incarcerated over a weekend pending court appearance the next Monday.

David contacted Joel, stating that he wanted to change therapists because he felt he was not making progress, especially after his arrest. David had had some prior contact with Joel because he had participated in a series of brief group therapy sessions ostensibly for anger management, and David thought that he had benefited from the solution-focused orientation. David met with Joel and a team behind the mirror for his first session.

J: Haven't seen you for two years or so. What are you doing to keep yourself busy?

D: Well, I'm a lot closer to getting my degree at the community college. I've been a dean's list student except for this semester. I got two Fs because I was in jail and couldn't take my final exams.

J: Well, that will do it. How long have you been going to community college?

D: I'm about three-quarters through. I'm taking computer information systems. I've never been arrested before, either.

J: Always new experiences—life's an adventure [both laugh]. So, you're taking computer information systems. How are you thinking that you want to use that or where to take it?

[David goes into a long explanation about his difficulties concentrating and the issues that this has caused him. During the monologue he mentions that he had dropped out before but "begged the college" to take him back.]

J: So you dropped out and went back? How did you do that?

D: I didn't tell them the truth; I didn't tell them that I dropped out because of my social phobia. I told her I was working with a psychiatrist developing their software. That part was true. I told her I got overconfident and thought we'd go into business.

J: What told you that you could go back—that you could get beyond the difficulties you had?

D: I arranged my courses so I could do the ones I felt comfortable about first. But the two courses I have difficulty with are the only ones left. So my back is to the wall.

J: Let's suppose you are able to do what you need to do to get through. What's after that?

D: I would like to be a technical writer. Write user manuals. It's something I can do out of my house. The other thing that got me depressed, most companies require you to be in the office for the first three months. When I get around people, I feel in danger. That made me lose hope.

J: So, how will you know that coming here to see me will be helpful to you?

D: For one thing, I have to stop going into a state of denial, blaming everyone for how I feel.

J: So if that changes, what will be different?

D: I wouldn't feel angry but would be thinking, "how can I relate to this person better?" That's part of my agoraphobia. I'm always thinking, "it's them, it's them." Then I don't want to go anywhere.

J: So, if I've got this right, if people got angry with you, you would be figuring out how to move things around and maybe relate to them better?

D: What I usually do is get angry.

J: So, what would you be doing instead of getting angry?

D: Being deft with people and not thinking so much if someone thinks poorly of me; I wouldn't be angry. I have a brother, Charles, who is a real politician.

J: Ah! What does Charles do that you want to do more of?

D: He relates a lot better to my mother than I do. I live with my mom. When Charles is up here, little stuff doesn't bother him like it does me. It doesn't affect his self-esteem. Like when she interrupts him when he's speaking. But I feel threatened by that.

J: So what would you be doing differently?

D: Instead of saying, "don't interrupt me when I'm speaking," maybe just not caring, letting her talk and then taking it up when she's done.

J: That's interesting. We've talked now about ten or fifteen minutes. I've interrupted you a couple of times. How are you able to do that here?

D: I didn't notice that. You don't seem to be looking down on me. I don't know why I think my mother does that—it's crazy. It's part of my agoraphobia. I was bullied when I was a kid, so I link it all to that.

The initial period with David was used to structure the meaning of therapy. Therapy is about possibilities. Possibilities stem from discussions of exceptions, future possibilities, and solution-building instead of problem exploration. Especially when the client has been seeped in problem-focused therapy, it requires patience and dogged determination on the part of the therapist to invite the client into a solution-building conversation. One way Joel does this is by turning problems into solutions. Two interchanges took place during these few initial minutes in which Joel asked David to consider alternatives to the problem picture.

Self-Esteem

Of special note is David's use of the term *self-esteem*. We have found this an interesting concept that has pervaded the life not only of clients, but of the general public as well. As in David's case, self-esteem has linguistically become a noun—we frequently use the term as something that we have or is contained somewhere inside of us, for example, "I have good/bad self-esteem." Having worked with many parents and their children, we commonly hear parents express that the goal of therapy is to help the child because he or she lacks self-esteem.

Thinking of self-esteem as a noun has implications for therapy. Within that context, the purpose of therapy is to somehow raise the client's self-esteem, and if that can happen, the problem(s) will be solved. Many clients are convinced that they cannot do anything about improving their lives until they are somehow imbued with better or more self-esteem (we are not sure whether self-esteem is quantitative, qualitative, or both). This is an interesting dilemma. Because problem-focused therapies serve to highlight problem(s), and therefore further co-construct the view of the client as dysfunctional (Miller, 1997), how will better or more self-esteem happen? This might explain why clients make limited progress and therapy becomes interminable—they are waiting to be filled with self-esteem because they view that as the cause of their problems. In SFBP, we have no assumptions or explanations about the causes of problems or about how problems may or may not relate to solutions.

Our own casual observations lead us to hypothesize that people appear to think and feel better about themselves when they accomplish something that is meaningful to them and/or significant others. We are curious what might change if we think of the language game of self-esteem as a verb: self-esteem as a process of achieving through actions. This might very well reorient therapy from the focus of clients and therapists to clients and their own life contexts, in which they essentially "do" self-esteem.

It Would Mean I Have Confidence in My Future

J: [Asks the miracle question.]

D: I don't know if this is the right answer . . .

J: Yours is the right answer.

D: If I'm driving and I'm at a red light, I wouldn't feel boxed in and threatened.

J: What would you be feeling instead?

D: I would be a little impatient like everyone else. I feel like everyone is a threat to me.

J: So you would notice that you would be a little impatient waiting for the light to change. Other than that, not much else.

D: Maybe even appreciate the chance to relax.

J: So, waiting for the light might actually be relaxing for you. So if that happened—you get in the car, you drive somewhere, you get to this light, and you find yourself a little more relaxed; you're able to tolerate that light—what difference would that make for you?

D: It would mean I could work. Apply for a job in computer systems. I could actually work in an office.

J: Would that be the first sign?

D: Absolutely.

J: If I were in traffic behind you and I didn't know it was you, what do you think I would see? This guy at the light having the start of his miracle day.

D: Nothing at all. You wouldn't notice anything—just another ordinary Joe. Right now, if someone tailgates me, I get angry and deliberately slow down.

de Shazer et al. (1986) wrote:

> No matter how awful and how complex the situation, a small change in one person's behavior can lead to profound and far-reaching differences in the behaviors of all persons involved. (p. 209)

Too often, clients and therapists set out together to solve the big problem and neglect to notice the possibilities that exist in small changes. As solution-focused therapists, we are attuned to constructing solutions from the details of small differences. The previous dialogue is a perfect example. David stated that after the miracle, he would be comfortable at a red light. This alone could be seen as minuscule and insignificant. Alternatively, Joel saw it as a possibility for engaging David in a conversation about differences. As a result, they created together a meaning of this event that went beyond just relaxing at a red light to include the possibilities of employment and a better future.

J: On this miracle day, what would be different about that?

D: I wouldn't have my whole self-esteem wrapped up in standing up to this guy. I wouldn't link it with being bullied in the past. I've built up this whole myth that it was all the other kids' fault that I was bullied when I was younger, and that had contributed to my agoraphobia at age twenty-two. If I could just realize you get what you give and treat other people well, they'll treat me well. Part of me understands that. But there's another part of me that doesn't.

J: The part of you that understands that, tell me about that part.

As therapists, we are constantly faced with choosing to which of the client's utterances we will respond. Our responses let the client know the rules of therapy—what we as therapists consider important and therefore where we want the client to focus his or her attention. As much as we might want our relationship with the client to be one of equality, we cannot avoid the client's view of us as having expertise. After all, why should clients see a therapist if by our training and experience we do not have something useful to offer them? As solution-focused therapists, we narrowly define our expertise as having knowledge of what in all probability will result in a useful conversation (Holmes & Cantwell, 1994).

We do not see that we are experts on clients and their lives or on problems and their causes and cures. We do see ourselves as experts on solution-building conversations, however. Narrowly defining our expertise allows us to be more open to listening and learning from clients about what is important to them and their strengths and resources. When we limit our area of expertise, we expand possibilities for the client.

Joel had two clear choices: (1) ask about the "agoraphobic" side of David or (2) ask about the other side. He had no guarantee that asking about either would result in something useful. Joel's own experience suggested that the latter choice provided a higher probability of success.

D: I'm afraid to let that be in the front seat; it's in the backseat.

J: When does that part come out?

D: When I was in jail for four days, I had to put my best foot forward in order to get along with the other inmates.

J: How did you do that?

D: I spent my time meditating. I had the intent of bringing out my Buddhist nature. I really meant it.

J: Jail kind of evoked that?

D: Yeah.

J: When the potential confrontations happened, what did you do to move it in another direction?

D: There was a young man who looked like more of a typical type of prisoner. I was doing the martial arts. I'm a second-degree black belt. I've been doing it since I was fifteen. He walked up to me and I didn't know what he was going to do. He was close to me. I was just about to start a form and he was standing right next to me. I said, "Excuse me, if you wouldn't mind, I just need a little space.

I'm just about to do a form." I just engaged him in a conversation. I wasn't used to his type and he wasn't used to my type but we both were prisoners—we both had the browns on. It wound up very positive. We talked for a while. I gave him an example of how to act like you're nuts so they'll put him in a mental hospital instead of prison. I had to bring out my better side in that situation.

J: I know you had to, but how did you do it?

D: The intent was there.

When Joel asked about the details of "the other side," David responded by relating his personal capacities and resources. It essentially served to reconstruct the jail experience as something potentially useful. We see our primary job as to co-construct something useful from whatever the client brings to the encounter. As Anderson and Goolishian (1992) stated,

> The "problems" dealt with in therapy can be thought of as emanating from social narratives and self-definitions that do not yield an agency that is effective for the task implicit in their self-narratives. Therapy provides opportunity for the development of new and different narratives that permit an expanded range of alternative agency for "problem" dis-solution. (p. 31)

J: In terms of the jail, how was the agoraphobia different?

D: I noticed it; it was there. I can look normal. It's all I can do to hold myself together. In jail, everything is simple. Jail is simple compared to being in an office for eight hours.

J: Coming back to this miracle day, what else would different?

Joel asked a question that he hoped would elicit a deconstructing response. If David had answered that in fact the "agoraphobia" had been different, it might have served to suggest that the problem is not constant and unchangeable and is therefore alterable. Instead, the response reestablished the problem as constant. Joel returned to the miracle question. Gale Miller (Miller & de Shazer, 1998) observed that devices such as the miracle question or scaling could be used as session anchors. When the conversation moves in a potentially less-than-useful direction, the therapist can always return to the miracle question to re-anchor the conversation toward solution talk.

D: I would be nice to my mother all day.

J: So what would she notice?

D: I'm not nitpicky. I'm not hypersensitive.

J: Not nitpicky, not hypersensitive; so, if I asked her, "What did you notice today about David that's different?" What would she say?

D: "He was nice to me all the time—considerate, kind, and appreciative."

J: Appreciative?

D: Recognize the small things that she does all the time.

J: What small things would you notice?

D: She buys the food and cooks.

J: How would that make a difference for her?

D: She would be getting what she's entitled to. I'm ashamed that I take my agoraphobia out on her.

J: So that's something you really want to change.

D: [Nods in agreement.]

As Joel patiently inquired about the details of difference, the desired outcomes for therapy became clearer and more realistic. Clients often come to therapy with vague and large expectations that are expressed as the absence of the problem. In David's case, he wanted to be rid of "his agoraphobia" that had plagued him since junior high school. In Stephen's case, he wanted to "get help with [his] schizophrenia." Although it was clear that David viewed the central problem as being "[his] agoraphobia" and, in fact, mentioned this frequently, the questions that Joel asked served to create a very different conversation regarding the details of difference. The results included very practical goals: holding down a job and improving the relationship with his mother. Similar to Haley (Miller, 1997), Joel did not let a seemingly unresolvable disorder be the problem. By reframing the situation as involving a job and relationships, Joel deconstructed agoraphobia, which has no solution, into something with solutions.

J: After the miracle happened, and you were more considerate, what would that mean to you—how would it be helpful to you?

D: For one thing, it would mean I was in control of myself. It would also mean I wasn't always focusing on the negative. It would mean I have confidence in my future. I can make a living. If I weren't overreacting to the small things, it would mean that the big things would work out.

J: As Mom sees you doing this, what would her reaction be?

D: She would be really happy because it would be easier for her every day. I think she would have more confidence in my future.

J: If your mom were here right now and I asked her what she's seeing that's telling her that you're moving in that direction, what do you think she would say? That she's proud of as your mom.

D: There were some things in the past that she can point to as signs of progress. I did work at a food distribution center for a year. That's great for someone with agoraphobia.

J: How were you able to do that?

D: I didn't want to be without financial resources. I was motivated—I wanted to get my degree.

If a solution is to be useful, it must be both possible and make a difference in the person's life. Of necessity, the results of the difference must be constructed within the client's own social context among those participating. Simon and Berg (1997) pointed out that

> As opposed to the medical model that assumes that problems are within the individual, SFBT contextualizes solutions socially. Solutions arise from the individual's social context and as a result of personal and social resources. (p. 118)

David expressed his desire to interact in different and hopefully more useful ways with his mother. Joel expanded the social context of change by asking how the mother would react when she began to notice the difference. Joel was curious whether the goal was realistic, so he asked an exception question. By answering David acknowledged that the goal was in fact possible.

I've Been Up to a Seven Before

J: If I had a scale, where ten is the day after the miracle, zero is maybe when you first went to jail, where would you put yourself on that scale?

D: I have to say a six. When I sent the threatening fax, I was probably at a five.

J: So, let's start with the six. What's the difference between six and zero?

D: Zero is when I have a fit of rage. One is when I first had agoraphobia and I had panic attacks. Two is I get despondent a couple times a month. Four is when I'm feeling calm but apathetic. Five, when I sent that fax, at least I was trying to deal with something—I did it the wrong way.

J: Five is at least you were motivated to try something.

D: Right. Six is that I learned from the experience that it's my responsibility how people react to me.

J: So, if I get this, six is that you recognized that you have some responsibility how people react to you. Like what you did with this guy in jail.

D: Yeah.

As in Stephen's case, we can again see how useful scaling is to explore exceptions to the problem. In David's case, it also served to show the progress that he already had made even before he saw Joel. Could these have been as a result of his previous therapy? The answer is certainly that elements of his conversations with his previous therapist were probably useful. All therapies, no matter the therapist's stated theoretical orientation, appear to have similar results (Beutler, Crago, & Arizmendi, 1986). Perhaps the difference is that Joel's focus is on co-constructing differences that make a difference.

J: How high do you think you could reach on that scale?

D: Consistently, eight.

J: How would you know that you were at eight?

D: I could hold a job. That would be eight.

J: What would be the signs that you could hold a job?

D: If I could sit in a computer lab with other students and concentrate on my work.

J: What makes you think that eight is even possible?

D: I've been up to a seven before.

J: So, seven is possible. What makes you think eight is possible?

D: I don't know. I hope it's possible.

J: If you were able to get to and stay around that seven consistently, would that be okay?

D: If it was enough to hold a job. If I had a job, I would have money and I would be able to socialize more.

It was not Joel's job to convince David that the goal was possible. It was David's job to convince himself that the goal was possible. David stated that 7 was possible because 7 had happened before. Although he was hopeful that his situation would go beyond 7 (whatever that might mean specifically for David), neither he nor we are certain that things could go even higher. The goal of therapy is not reaching 10. Rather, the goal is reaching a place where the client has developed a satisfactory solution to the problem. This is why Joel asked whether 7 would be satisfactory. The attempt (and hopefully effect) was to imply that therapy is brief and should address what is likely—not necessarily ideal. Therapy, especially brief therapy, can be viewed as a good enough beginning, one that the client will be able to continue on his or her own (Simon & Berg, 2004).

J: Let's suppose our conversation here is helpful to you in some small way. In the course of the week, something happens that moves you in a positive way. When you return, you tell me that you're at seven on the scale. What would be happening that moved you up that one point on the scale?

D: If I really had a different attitude toward my mother. That would mean I have more confidence deep down inside that things will work out.

J: If you brought a video of this happening with no sound, what would we see?

D: Calmer, slower, nicer facial expression. She'd be smiling more because she wouldn't be having her feelings hurt.

J: If she were happier, what would that mean to you?

D: The other thing is if I were doing my computer studies more. I've been slowing down; I think it may be depression.

J: Okay, which one would most likely happen first, the changes with Mom or the computer studies?

D: I would say the thing with Mom because the emotional content has to change.

J: One last scale: In terms of your willingness to put in the hard work, if ten were as long as it's legal, didn't cost you much, and no one gets hurt, you'd be willing to try any crazy idea we might come up with. Zero is the opposite. Where would you put yourself?

D: Nine. I say that because we all have weak moments.

J: Great. A lot of good information. So I'm going to meet with the team.

[Joel returns after consulting with the team.]

J: They had a lot to say about you. We were really impressed at your willingness to work this way. You really seem to be motivated to change. You seem to have an understanding of yourself. The other thing that's remarkable is that you've had these awful things that have happened to you—you've ended up in jail—you're smart about learning from these situations. You have a clear picture of where you want to go.

We were thinking about the problem that you presented here. We have a couple of thoughts about that. It's hard to find the balance with integrity. On one hand, we had the sense that you have a lot of self-respect and integrity. And then this politician thing. Hard to figure out how you'd be the politician and at the same time maintain your integrity. It seems to be important to you to be true to yourself. It's important for you to feel respected. The team thought you found this field that you know a lot about, that excites you. You were smart to find the direction that motivates you.

What comes through to us is that you really care about Mom. It says something about your motivation that Mom is important in motivating you to do better. It says something that when given the choice, you said that Mom would notice the change first.

We were impressed with what you've done in difficult situations. We talked about what happened to you in the jail. We couldn't imagine how horrible that must be; have your freedom taken away, to be put in jail surrounded by these people with guards in your face. And yet you were able to hold it together. We had a laugh about teaching the other prisoner about how to act nuts. It seems you've spent all those years in mental health and they've paid off in some way [both laugh]. You taught someone how to be crazy.

I'm not sure you're going to see it this way; it seemed to us that you have these insights about pacing yourself. When things become too much, you don't go further than you're willing to go or able to go at that point. Sometimes you need to wait until you are ready. Something to think about.

D: I always looked at that as a negative.

J: The other thing we were really impressed with: a lot of people who have been in therapy for a long time, they think big. You were able to focus on the small steps that for you will make a difference. For example, by changing your relationship with your mom, you can have an effect in other areas in your life. We thought about this idea that you have that by changing your reaction to other people, they will change toward you. We would be interested to hear as you test this out, how it makes a difference for you and what you learn. We talked about what's normal and what's not normal. It seems to us it's normal to use your skills. It seems normal to us that you want to have good relationships with people. It seems normal to us that you want to get ahead in life. There are a lot of these things you do that seem pretty normal to us. We have a suggestion: It sounds like you're really moving in some nice ways. We thought maybe we could give you a way of focusing that even more. Pick a day, pick it the night before. Go to sleep and act as if while you were sleeping, the miracle happened. Spend the next day acting as if the miracle happened. Notice what's different.

David identified his diagnosis as a part of himself: "my agoraphobia." This could lead only to the conclusion that agoraphobia was an intrinsic part of him and therefore was incurable. As long as he "had" agoraphobia, he would be spending his time trying to figure out how to get rid of it. Similarly, Stephen stated that he "is schizophrenic." de Shazer (1998) observed, "Our grammar leads us naturally to the conclusion that schizophrenia is incurable. Once a schizophrenia, always a schizophrenia [*sic*]" (p. 2). The team began the process of deconstructing David's view of himself as having agoraphobia. They pointed out all the things that he did that could be viewed as normal, and recommended a between-session suggestion that challenged him to see beyond his diagnosis.

Second Session

J: You've been in therapy for a long time. I want to make sure that what we do is making a difference. What is it that's happened since the last time I saw you that lets you know that transferring here was probably a good idea?

Joel's initial question served to orient David in three important ways: (1) therapy is about having conversations that ultimately make a difference in the client's life, (2) the focus of that difference is in the client's life outside of the therapy office, and (3) the therapist is interested in a conversation about what David noticed that made a positive difference in his life.

D: I tried to have a miracle yesterday and the thing is, the miracle happened Monday night. Something that's extremely rare—it's happened once or twice before. I pissed myself off about my mother. I expressed my frustration calmly just the way I'm talking now.

J: To your mom?

D: Yeah

J: Wow!

D: I haven't always been able to do that. That was the only time I was angry at my mother since last time we met. I handled myself with control. It was better than keeping it in. I expressed my frustration to her calmly and that let it out.

EMOTIONS IN THERAPY

Ever since Freud theorized that psychopathology is the result of the build up of repressed negative emotions, decathexis has long been the staple of clinical theory and practice (Bushman, 2002). The concept has seeped into our culture as evidenced by popular and overused expressions such as "letting it out" and "venting." What we find interesting is how the metaphorical nature of emotions has become concretized. It is as if feelings are viewed as substances that actually take up space somewhere "deep" in the person. This is especially true of negative emotions, which seem for some reason (maybe their specific gravity is greater) to push out the positive emotions. Or, maybe because positive emotions are lighter, they do not seem to go as deeply. Regarding the treatment of emotions in general by therapists, Miller and de Shazer (2000) stated,

> We argue that therapists have constructed a professional field of emotions that treats emotions as abstract entities about which some therapists are uniquely knowledgeable and perhaps even

experts. Clients may display emotions, but only therapists understand what emotions "really" mean. (p. 7)

What appears to happen is that negative emotions build up within us, and untoward consequences occur at the point that they take up too much space. From David's statements, we might infer that the build up of negative emotions resulted in an exacerbation of his agoraphobia, and this in turn caused a concomitant rage, which then was directed at his mother.

Within the language game of emotions as concrete objects, the job of the therapist is to provide the outlet for emotions so that they need not build up. The analogy is that of a pressure cooker for which the therapist is the valve that releases the pressure. What reinforces this concept is that when most people see a therapist to "vent," they often in fact leave feeling better (although most clients will admit that this improvement is very short lived). The logical conclusion is that venting resulted in altered emotions when in fact it may have been that the substance of the conversation helped the client perceive the situation in a more positive and hopeful way.

Miller and de Shazer (2000) further stated,

> Anger, love, hate and grief are activities that we do, that others may observe us doing, and we may observe them doing. We also stress how emotions are aspects of concrete social contexts, and how their meanings vary across social contexts. Viewed from this standpoint, emotions are not a separate domain of social life or a distinctive field for therapist specialization and expertise. (p. 7)

Therapists and clients have many interactions during the course of a conversation that offer alternative language games that may have beneficial results. Joel's response with David was to focus on the differences rather than the emotions.

I'm Ready for Things to Happen

J: So, what did she notice different about you that time?

D: She must have seen I wasn't losing my temper. She must have seen that, absolutely.

J: How much less rare would this need to happen for her to go, "something's going on with David here."

D: Maybe two times out of three—even that's not good enough. Maybe eventually nine times out of ten. And even the exception would have to be different. Throwing things has to be gone completely.

J: How did you do it?

D: First of all, when anything changes favorably in my life, I feel more hopeful. I regard this as a better therapy situation. Also, I went to a Buddhist meeting and did chanting with other people. I think just being with other people gives me more of a positive attitude.

J: What's the relationship between that and how you were able to deescalate with your mom?

D: I think going to the meeting and getting something out of that, having a change of therapy, which I regard as having more potential, made me feel more hopeful about the future. When I'm doing something to improve now, I'm not so angry about the past. It's more water under the bridge.

During the course of the conversation, David realized that as he was beginning to think more positively of the future, he found himself less angry about the past. Furthermore, he was the subject as well as the object of the change. Of course, we cannot know for certain, but we can at least speculate that the first session served to reorient David from that which is unchangeable ("my agoraphobia") to that which has already changed: different therapy, going to meetings, and a significantly improved way of expressing his anger to his mother. Taking the first step toward doing something differently is doing something differently. The therapist can enhance this difference in the dialogue with the client. Simply punctuating the effort itself as a difference is likely to move the client toward a "difference that makes a difference" (Bateson, 1972, p. 453). Joel's questions focused David on what was making a difference and how.

J: So, when you see possibilities, you dwell less on the things in the past.

D: I think so.

J: As you had this conversation with your mom, what was Mom's reaction; what did she do?

D: She was listening to what I had to say. What is more important was that she wasn't getting upset.

J: Let's see if I get this: she wasn't as worried about what your reaction was going to be?

D: Right. She saw that it wasn't going to escalate, so she was calm. Because I was calm.

J: How did her calmness affect you?

D: I never thought about it. The fact is when I overreact, that gets her anger up. Then I react with anger and it just gets worse. But that didn't happen.

J: That's a rarity for her I suppose.

D: Yeah, she's entitled to that all the time. At least it happened once. I think I need to internalize that more.

J: What would be the sign for you that you internalized that more, or at least started that process?

D: I think that I held my temper this time. That was very difficult for me, but it just happened. I don't know exactly why it happened, it just did.

J: What is it that tells you this is the beginning of a new direction for you?

D: It helped for me to be determined that I was going to have a miracle. As a matter of fact, the next time I was calm as well—a little lethargic, but calm.

J: What tells you that what you did with Mom is the start of something that you are going to be doing more often rather than something rarely here and there?

D: I need to do this every day. I have to pretend that I'm better. You said to wake up and pretend that my agoraphobia was gone. And all the spin-off effects: low social life, low incomes are no longer there. Actually, the next day, I felt very lethargic but also able to appreciate little things I usually overlook. It was hard work. I didn't get much done the next day.

J: So which is more hard work? That or just letting it go?

D: There's much more cost being angry. Maybe I just wasn't used to being calm.

J: What would help getting to that three out of four times—nine out of ten times eventually?

D: Well, I think that when this court issue is resolved, that will help. I need to change my financial bottom line. I don't want to live on disability all my life. I want to become a technical writer. [Dave relates how he has tried to apply for disability benefits without much success.] I have to recapture my confidence that I'm going to be a success in the future and be a technical writer or programmer.

Joel accepted what David said without challenge because he had learned to respect clients' ideas, even when they seem unrelated to the goal. Miller (1997) said the following:

> Accepting surface appearances is also one way in which solution-focused therapists display respect for their clients, and utilize clients' resources in defining and remedying their troubles. (pp. 66-67)

This set of transactions between Joel and David is a clear example of the results of what happens when the therapist patiently asks about the details of differences. This is a very different picture from the one of David who had been in therapy for many years, had an intransigent mental illness, and who complained of making very little progress. This expansive picture began with the observation from David that he had one set of more positive transactions with his mother during which he was able to express his anger without escalation.

The interaction between David and Joel can be understood from a poststructural language game. To again cite Miller (1997),

> Poststructuralists offer a very different view of language. They treat social realities as constructed and sustained through our use of language, and emphasize the ways in which our thoughts are shaped by the words that we use. (p. 66)

Essentially, Joel and David engaged in a series of transactions in which together they deconstructed David as agoraphobic and reconstructed David as Buddhist, martial artist, successful college student, and future technical writer or programmer.

J: What would be the first signs that you are starting to regain a little bit of confidence in the future?

D: Well, I've been learning what I need to, but at a snail's pace. I think it's the result of my agoraphobia. If I were picking up the pace a little more, that would give me more confidence. In the last couple of weeks, I have been pushing myself more.

J: Really? Pushing yourself more. What do you mean?

D: I've been working on programming.

J: What's made the difference for you that you've speeded things up?

D: I've got to use this court thing as a springboard—changing the negative into positive. I can make it a turning point. I've been trying to get everything in sync.

J: So, what would need to happen for what happened with Mom on Monday to happen more often?

D: A couple of things: If I worked more on my computer studies. If I speeded up and treated it like a job, then I would have hope. Also, a few months ago I adopted a dog from the humane society. When I went there to get the dog, there was a very attractive girl there, Sally. I didn't give it much thought. I got something in the mail— an invitation to a reunion picnic for anyone who adopted a dog or cat. Sally had signed it that she would like to see the dog and me there. With my agoraphobia, normally I wouldn't even consider it; there will be a lot of people there and it'll be very open. But I'm going to do it. The other thing is that the local town is giving a karate demonstration. I might volunteer to help out by giving a demonstration.

J: That's amazing. What tells you you're ready to do this?

D: I don't have much to lose. If I look a little nervous, so what? I don't think I'll have a panic attack. My martial arts training gives me pretty good control physically.

J: So, it sounds like what is really helpful to you is keeping hope for the future [David nods in agreement]. If I had a scale, ten is incredibly hopeful and zero is the opposite, where would you put yourself?

D: I'd have to say between seven and eight—a little higher than last time.

J: What accounts for the difference?

D: The fact that I controlled my temper with my mom. And I talked to my lawyer and it looks like the whole court thing will be resolved. I think also that I decided to challenge this dog and cat fest; I'm going to go.

J: How would you know that you had moved up just a little bit more, maybe to a solid eight?

D: Well, if I can do the same thing with my mom the next couple of times.

J: Is that just a small amount or is that much higher?

D: I think it's possible, because when things happen that are better, I have a better sense of progress. I'm ready for things to happen.

The conversation structured hope and expectation for a better future. At the same time, Joel asked questions that co-constructed the future as possible.

J: One more scale before I take a break. In terms of your confidence that you could go at least another step on that scale, where are you?

D: Based on my positive reaction to this invitation—that I decided I'm not going to let my agoraphobia stand in the way—I'd have to say seven and a half. The bottom line is this agoraphobia and anger that's ninety percent of everything for me.

J: In terms of things getting better, which do you think will likely get better first, the agoraphobia or the anger?

D: I see them as parallel. Both will happen at the same time. I saw a psychologist once in school who said that agoraphobia is anger turned inward. What do you think about that?

J: There are all kinds of theories. But that's what they are, theories. Let's see if the team has any ideas about that.

J: [Returns from consulting with the team.] They first wanted to acknowledge the hard work that you've been doing. It seems to be paying off.

D: Thank you.

J: You've realized that you are the one who has control over your own behavior. There are some things that you just do that work, not the least your Buddhist orientation. That really seems to be a compass for you. Your karate: the sense we have is you understand the spirit. We like your idea that each day for you could be a miracle.

You can have small miracles every day. You took that from our suggestion and made it your own. That was exciting for us.

Wow, what happened with your mom? That's remarkable. It seemed to us that the hard work you're doing is moving in new directions. You're experimenting with different behaviors. You see yourself differently and you're seeing your future differently. We talked about the humane society picnic and how that's different for you. We wondered what she saw about you that got her to write that note saying she hoped to see you there.

The team talked about the lethargy that you talked about and thought that what you said made a lot of sense. One of the team members recalled that when she goes on vacation, she spends the first couple of days just letting down, sitting on a lounge chair by the beach, just not moving. It sounds like this may be one of those good lethargies. You were putting in a lot of hard work, and maybe this was one of those times to just let down and savor some of what you've done.

We thought about what you're doing here, what's the goal. What made sense is that you're making the rarities common place. You're taking the exceptions and making them the rules.

D: Yeah.

J: We thought how smart it is for you to see the issues with the court as a springboard and a turning point for you. You could have just as easily seen it the other way.

D: Sure.

J: You said the last panic attack was about eighteen years ago. We were curious about how many years after the last one does it take before you kind of not define yourself in that way anymore?

During the course of their conversation, the team suggested taking a risk and suggesting to David a deconstruction of the diagnosis. They reasoned that a number of positive events were happening in his life, he was feeling more confident in his progress, and he himself stated that he was ready to move beyond the label.

D: I still feel a lot of tension, though.

J: Sure.

D: But, yeah, a good point.

J: You know that it's the small steps that count. You seem to be doing two general things that are important: The first is that you create the future by first creating a vision of the future. The second is to know that success builds upon success. The only suggestion we have at this point is to notice what moves you up just that one point on the scale. If you want to move up higher, no extra charge.

D: [Laughs] I just wanted to say how this feedback has been affecting me. I have been learning how to handle my mother and other people—even my own internal dialogue—through this. The way you guys do this: instead of focusing on, "you don't do this right, you don't do that right," which would be true, you compliment me on what I'm doing right even if it's not a dominant part of me. That's how I should try to get what I want from other people. I have to handle my mother the way you handle me.

J: Well, that would be a neat experiment.

The progress that David made within the week between sessions is nothing short of remarkable. David returned for his fourth appointment with Joel and the team two weeks later. He continued talking about the progress he had been making and, in fact, referred to himself as having "mild agoraphobia." Joel took his customary break to consult with the team, and when he returned, he offered David the following suggestion:

J: We had this crazy idea. Each morning, toss a coin. If it comes up heads, act as if this mild agoraphobia has gone away; if tails, have your normal day. At the end of the day, note what's different. Do it as many days as you need until you've learned something from it. We would be interested in what you learn.

It Doesn't Have to Be the Central Part of My Life

David returned for his fifth session two weeks later.

D: The homework said, "Pretend that you don't have agoraphobia." You know what was really amazing? I didn't really make any life-style choices that were really different. I'm a very solitary type person. The stuff I did was the same as when I still had agoraphobia, so to speak. I like computing. I like walking in the woods with my German shepherd. I like being on the Web. I like martial arts. I like military miniatures. Nothing changed really.

J: So what did that kind of insight mean to you?

D: I kept thinking about what you said during our second session. You said, "Isn't it time you stop defining yourself as someone who has agoraphobia? You haven't had a panic attack since 1980." I felt the agoraphobia was no longer the center of my life. It's something big in my left flank or my right flank. It's not small, not negligible; but it's not formidable—it doesn't have to be the central part of my life.

J: How did you move it from the center to the right flank or the left flank?

D: By pretending that I was someone who didn't have agoraphobia. I didn't avoid anything that I wanted to do. Of course, I don't avoid most things anyway—if I want to do it, I do it.

J: So, you're a guy with agoraphobia who does what he wants to when he wants to. How do you do that?

D: Yeah; someone once told me that the definition of agoraphobia is avoidance. Ah!

J: Don't most people avoid what they don't have to do and they do it if they have to do it? I don't like paying bills but I eventually have to pay them if I want to keep a roof over my house. So what did you learn from it?

D: My fundamental definition of myself is not someone who has agoraphobia. Maybe it's a peripheral aspect of my life. Therefore, there's no reason why I can't reclaim my self-esteem. [He tells a story that he politely confronted a neighbor and felt good about it. Joel asks him what that meant to him.]

D: I've been feeling better about myself and more equal. I'm not thinking about myself as an agoraphobic, fundamentally. It's just one aspect of myself. It's not my definition of myself. My core is me. I kept defining myself as someone with agoraphobia as if that was my core. This exercise I did over the last few weeks helped me. I started out pretending I didn't have agoraphobia. What I realized is that my life is largely independent of that. I can permit myself to be happy.

J: So you can permit yourself to be happy.

D: Yeah. I may need a little practice. It might have to be deliberate for a little while.

J: What does Mom notice?

D: I didn't have any violent episodes. I got testy several times, but not in a major way, not shouting, not in an abusive way. It was minor.

J: How did that happen; what was the difference there?

D: Well, part of my environment. The court thing is resolving itself and VESID [Vocational and Educational Services for Individuals with Disabilities] is getting started. Part of it was internal. I'm reclaiming my life. It's like a declaration of independence in a sense. It started out as role-playing but I'm not in a straitjacket because of this agoraphobia. It's just one aspect of me. Also, I was not only less obnoxious, but I was nice more often.

J: Oh, so that's different.

D: One time something happened and it was like a miracle. We got into a spontaneous conversation. She was trying to encourage me. She said, "You think you have problems." She said she had a terrible childhood; her parents separated three times. She then told me something I never knew. Her parents refused to come to her wedding. I spontaneously hugged her. She almost started crying. I realized that I touched something in her and I need to do that more often.

J: So, who was more shocked about that, you or she?

D: I think that I was.

J: That you realized you could do that, have that reaction?

D: It's been so long since I expressed genuine sympathy—from the gut. It was that I was no longer feeling so empty that I couldn't give.

J: So a scale where ten is on track, where would you put yourself?

D: Eight.

J: How come eight?

D: Things in my environment are coming together: I'm going to get back to school one way or another. I'm starting to feel better about myself. But that's work I'm doing internally. I'm declaring independence from this agoraphobia. I'm not going to define myself as agoraphobia. That's just a small blemish.

J: Where do you think Mom would put you?

D: Six and a half.

J: So, up there. Is nine possible?

D: Because of what's happening in my environment, I have to say yes. Of course that's not the ideal. I should be able to go to nine internally.

J: How would you know that you were at nine?

D: If I come home from rush hour traffic and don't have a wave of irritability.

J: What makes you think it's possible that it can happen?

D: Because I'm getting in control of my life both because of my environment coming together and because I'm having this new insight since starting here. Agoraphobia and me are not synonymous. I've said that intellectually before, but now I'm really starting to feel it.

J: Let me meet with the team.

[Joel returns.]

J: We're really impressed with a number of profound things you said. You said that everything doesn't need to be complicated. You need to take action and do it in increments. We have nothing to add to that; we'll just let that stand because it's incredibly profound.

You are not your agoraphobia. It's just an aspect of yourself. It seems to us you see that as not central but right or left flank, other things are taking its place. It allows you to use the energy in other ways. Our sense is your creativity has gone up. You're permitting yourself to be successful. It's not that it wasn't there; it always existed. You just gave yourself permission to find it. In the same way, you've taken the suggestions we gave you and created them in your own way to make them work for you.

The other aspect of that energy is your openness to options. You're much more open to your own happiness. Of course it takes practice, but the way you're thinking about yourself is rapidly changing. You said you're declaring your independence from agoraphobia; you're reclaiming your own life. You're allowing your own spontaneity to come out.

It really touched us that you had that spontaneous empathy for your mother. You really understood her. For that one moment you were no longer son and mother but two adults. You said you shouldn't let external forces make you happy; it should be internal. It's hard for us to know the difference. You don't create the external forces—they exist. When you're ready to take them in, you take them in.

We have another suggestion for you. Since the last suggestion was helpful to you, we suggest you do it again, but change it a
little bit. Flip a coin each evening. If it's heads, deliberately allow
yourself to be happy. Think about it. If it's tails, let it happen spontaneously.

D: Okay. So if it's heads permit myself to be happy.

J: Deliberately.

D: Yes. And if it's tails, just let it happen—interesting.

Joel and the team worked with David for a total of eight sessions
over a period of nine months. David continued to report improvements:

- He moved into his own apartment.
- The number of "explosive episodes" with his mother decreased
  significantly to about once a month, and David reported that
  when they did occur, they were "minor."
- He stated that he was "thinking more creatively," and as a result
  he no longer felt "depressed."
- He returned to the community college and began his computer
  studies once again.

I Never Had a Chance to Talk Myself into Anything Worse

One of the team members interviewed David about his experiences
at his last session with Joel and the team.

Q: What happened here that was helpful?

D: I didn't focus on my problems. I didn't talk myself into reinforcing
my problems. Getting the feedback helped. When it's feedback time,
I'm apprehensive. After years of giving myself negative feedback,
I drank up good feedback—it encouraged me more.

Q: Is there anything that we didn't do well, we missed, or need to do
better?

D: This is dramatically different from what I had before. This is much
better, at least for me. It's such an enormous difference; I can't find
anything wrong with it. It jump starts a positive cycle. I never had a
chance to talk myself into anything worse.

Q: How were the arrangements for you, the team, and the camera?

D: It might have been a little more difficult for me than other people. It was good for me. Once I was talking to Joel, it didn't matter.

Q: You get to scale Joel. On a scale of zero to ten, how helpful was Joel?

D: Well, I wouldn't give anyone more than nine. God is ten. I would give Joel a nine.

Q: What puts him there?

D: He did get me talking about small steps. He concentrated on progress rather than the problem. He ran the session. If I ran the session, like I did in the previous therapy, I run the session and do all the talking. I have an audience instead of a therapist. How am I going to change? I didn't mind Joel running the session. He knows his stuff and I respect someone who knows his stuff.

Q: If you go home today and a friend or family member asked you about therapy, how would you describe what happened here?

D: It was like something outside of me drawing out something inside of me. What makes me better is what's inside of me. A good influence can draw it out. If I don't have something to draw it out, it might just stay asleep. It's a good influence.

Q: Were the between-session suggestions helpful to you? And if so, which ones specifically?

D: They were helpful because it made it tangible. For example, role-playing like you never had agoraphobia. The other was try making yourself happy and then be happy spontaneously. It made it concrete. It takes it from philosophy to practical.

Q: Would you recommend that a friend or family member come here if they thought therapy would be helpful to them?

D: Yes, I would.

CONCLUSION

de Shazer et al. (1986) stated,

> The task of Brief Therapy is to help clients do something different, by changing their interactive behavior and/or their interpretation of behavior and situations so that a solution (a resolution of their complaint) can be achieved. (p. 108)

Clients who have been inductees in the mental health system for many years have become their diagnoses. Most often with such clients, progress can be made when they begin to deconstruct how they think of themselves as disabled and restructure their self-view as "abled." The job of the therapist therefore is to use questions to challenge the way clients have come to think about themselves, others, and the contexts of their lives.

Too often, mental health professionals shrug their shoulders and blame clients for a lack of progress. We have developed a lexicon of attributes that maintain the view of such a client: "resistant," "in denial," "noncompliant," and "borderline" to name just a few. In his article, "The Death of Resistance," de Shazer (1984) wrote,

> Therefore, the therapist's stance is not *if* change will occur, but rather *when,* or *where,* or *what type of* changing will occur [italics in original]. A concept of "resistance" within this framework would hinder and handicap the therapist because it implies that change is not inevitable, setting up a contest between changing and nonchanging. (pp. 16-17)

The co-constructed process of restructuring proved itself as powerful for David when he came to think that "my agoraphobia" might be just one aspect of himself. We often think that in order for therapy to be successful, its complexity must match or be greater than the complexity of the problem(s). Yet in David's case, it was the simple foci on what he wanted, what was possible, his resources and abilities (versus disabilities), and his road map to the future that made the difference. We create difference when we have different conversations than those that have kept people locked in the mental health system for years.

Chapter 6

Rethinking the Medical Model

A DIFFERENT LANGUAGE GAME

In the capacity of treatment coordinator at Fairview Psychiatric Center,[1] Joel observed the following interaction between a staff member and an adolescent hospitalized at the center. The adolescent group at the time was involved in daily education classes. This particular individual had been in an altercation with the teacher and was ordered by the teacher to return to the unit. The teenager initially argued her point and then was escorted from the room by a hospital staff member. Once in the hall, the adolescent again argued that the situation was unfair. The staff member replied that the adolescent had to learn how to respect adults and accept the consequences of her actions, and that her behaviors were evidence of her psychiatric issues. The adolescent in turn insisted that no one understood her and then repeated her mantra, "it's not fair."

The dialogue continued with each party insisting on its point of view, the volume increasing with each interaction. Simultaneously, the staff member moved closer to the adolescent whose back literally was to the wall. At a critical moment, the staff member was in close approximation to the teenager, waving her finger, pointing directly at the teen and repeating in a loud voice that as part of the girl's treatment she needed to show respect for adults. Other staff members of the hospital began to gather around in expectation that the adolescent's behavior would escalate. On cue, the adolescent lashed out at the staff member and the other staff intervened, holding the teenager and taking her to the floor as she loudly screamed and struggled. She was returned forcibly to her room and placed on "one-on-one"—confined to her room with 24-hour staff supervision.

Solution-Focused Brief Practice
© 2007 by The Haworth Press, Taylor & Francis Group. All rights reserved.
doi:10.1300/5507_06

In the "psychological autopsy" the next day, the incident was reviewed and the child's behaviors were characterized as "going off," a common term used by treatment staff for interpreting adolescent angry behaviors. The team discussed the behavior as consistent with the child's psychopathology and diagnosis. The psychiatrist suggested an increase in medication to help the adolescent better control her angry impulses. Staff also decided that, as part of the treatment plan, they needed to be consistent in their dealings with the teenager so that she could learn better anger management and respect for "authority figures."

This story serves well to demonstrate the difference between making meaning of behaviors within the medical model versus viewing behaviors as inseparable from their social contexts. Within the medical model, behaviors are theorized as motivated by internal processes that usually exist outside the awareness of the individual and are pathological. Treatment becomes focused on helping individuals name, understand, and ultimately control their impulses.

Wittgenstein's (1958) use of the term *language games* may be useful in describing this scenario. Briefly, language games are how we make meaning of words with others in conversations through the structures (grammar and patterns) within which the words exist. They also include the behaviors that accompany the meanings and words. Different language games result in very different outcomes, and when two people use different language structures, confusing communication usually results.

In the previous description, the child's behaviors were seen by the staff as part of a medical language game. The teen was operating within a different language game, one we might call, "Life isn't fair and adults are out to get me!" Her behavior made sense to her within a context of attempting to convince adults of her position. Thus, she escalated her attempts to reason with them. The staff, however, placed the behavior within a context of the girl's mental or behavioral disorder and thus saw it as more evidence of the disorder. Consistent with that language game, the social context of the behaviors were considered irrelevant by the staff because the adolescent's actions were assumed to be a result of intrapsychic processes. The altercation between the adolescent and the staff member was therefore understood as consistent with the child's psychopathology. This inevitably resulted in a treatment plan that dictated increased medication and clin-

ical intervention intent upon improving the adolescent's ego process-
ing functions.

More important, if the adolescent "complied" with the recommendations, she ultimately risked defining herself as disabled and dysfunctional, thus continuing the induction into a lifelong role as long-
term user of mental health services. This is, of course, unless the
adolescent is imbued with the ability to resist, in which case she is
then described as in denial, noncompliant, and/or resistant, which in
turn would necessitate increased effort to convince her of the reality
of her medical condition so that she might be more amenable to treatment. Consistent with this language game, the hospital staff would
need to be increasingly alert to signs of the teenager's dysfunctional
behaviors and dutifully note these in her chart so that they would be
able to eventually confront her and break through her denial.

Inherent within this language game is the understanding that psychiatric conditions are stubbornly persistent and minimally alterable
only with long-term treatment and possible use of psychiatric medi-
cation(s). Such an understanding originates from the theoretical assumption that problematic behaviors mirror "deeper," inner psychic
processes. It logically follows from this argument that treatment
options are limited.

If the language game changes from one that attempts to explain
why individuals behave in the ways that they do to one that simply de-
scribes the behaviors within social contexts, the end results ultimately are different. Seeing behaviors as parts of interactions within
contexts inevitably increases the possibilities for intervention: many
parts of the context, not just intrapsychic pathology, can be the focus
of change. Of course, clients usually are the ones who must start the
change, but in a solution-focused language game, therapists are part
of the relational context and therefore can change their way of doing
things, which requires different responses from clients. Clients may
then be able to see their behaviors in context with others' behaviors
and think of ways that different behaviors on their part may elicit different behaviors on the part of others. A collaborative relationship
stands a better chance of including discussions around what can be
different than one that focuses on what the individual is doing wrong.
The difference is working *with* rather than *on* the client. The solution-
focused therapist looks for ways to invite the client to consider new
perspectives or behaviors that will better serve the client's needs,

rather than acting as an expert who knows exactly what the client should do and what the effects of doing that will be.

Figures 6.1 and 6.2 represent alternative scenarios: a medical language game and a solution-building language game. It is clear that interventions driven by solution-focused assumptions present a number of possible alternatives of co-constructing something useful from the

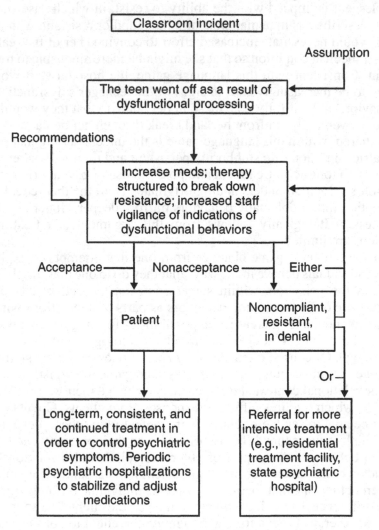

FIGURE 6.1. Medical Language Game

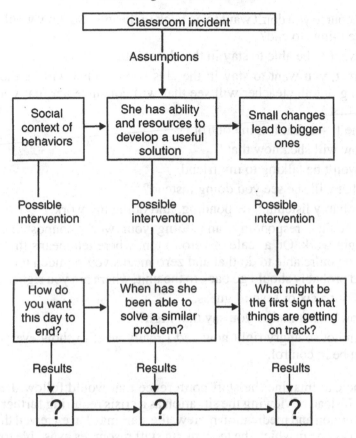

FIGURE 6.2. Solution-Building Language Game

episode. The solution-focused therapist utilizes a situation as an opportunity for learning, growth, and change. Taking just one of the interventions driven by a solution-focused assumption, the scenario would most likely have very different results from those described earlier:

ADOLESCENT (A): It's not fair, there were other people talking, she was singling me out!

STAFF (S): Right, it's not fair. Is it okay if we sit and talk about it?

A: Yeah, I don't want to go back to the unit, it's not fair.

S: Of course you don't want to go back to the unit. So, how would you like things to end?

A: I want to be able to stay in the classroom.

S: Great, you want to stay in the classroom. What will be the first thing that the teacher will see that will convince her that you can do that?

A: She'll see that I'm in control.

S: How will she know that?

A: I won't be talking to my friend.

S: What will she see you doing instead?

A: Probably listening, responding, and doing my work.

S: Listening, responding, and doing your work; sounds like that might work. On a scale of zero to ten, where ten means that right now you're able to do that and zero means you're much too angry and probably should go back to the unit, where are you right now?

A: About a six or seven I guess.

S: Wow! What makes you say that high?

A: I'm not so angry right now and I really want to show everyone I can be in control.

One can imagine the staff conference that would follow the episode. Instead of viewing the situation as a crisis requiring further staff intervention and medication review, the staff may have viewed the situation as one in which the teen, using staff resources, was able to gain control. The feedback to the adolescent from staff would have positively reinforced her ability to maintain control and to work constructively to find adaptive solutions.

This is just one possible intervention of many, each with the capacity to produce a positive result. Figure 6.2 represents the possible assumptions and interventions inherent within a solution-focused language game.

In contrast to the corresponding medical language game, the solution-focused language game could be represented as follows:

Descriptions of behaviors and events

Child is asked to leave in presence of peers; she refuses.

Solution-focused assumption 1

> Child's behaviors make sense in her social context: need to save face, exert autonomy.

Possible interventions for assumption 1

1. What does teenager want to be different?
2. How does she want this day to end?
3. Who might be surprised by how she might get herself back on track?
4. What might her parents say when they hear how she was able to develop a new way of responding when she is angry?

Solution-focused assumption 2

> She has the ability, capacity, and resources to develop a useful solution to the problem.

Possible interventions for assumption 2

1. When has she had a time that she was able to respond to a similar situation in a more useful way?
2. What will help her to turn the situation around?
3. Where is she on a scale of 0 to 10, in which 10 is although she is angry, she is confident that she can prove to everyone that she can interact in a helpful way, and 0 is that she needs to return to her room?

Although not exhaustive, the descriptions provide some idea of the increased possibilities that exist in a solution-focused language game. The assumptions can be used in combination throughout conversations. If one assumption does not lead to an intervention that creates a potentially useful result, another intervention can be tried. Given the vast number of possible interventions in combination with various assumptions, a high probability exists that some conversation will co-construct a positive resolution.

The probability that the conversation will result in a useful outcome increases because solution-focused practice is based on descriptions of solutions that have worked in the past for the particular client. In contrast, the medical model assumes only one solution to a psychiatric problem exists, which arises from the understanding of the ultimate causes of psychopathology (de Shazer, 1985), and which is applied to everyone. If that intervention does not help, the medical model language game (e.g., different medications, different therapies) all too often ends in blaming the client for the therapy's failure. Solutions that have worked for other clients may be attempted, but it is not typical to use the client's own exceptions and solutions.

SOLUTION-BUILDING CONVERSATIONS

During Joel's tenure at Fairview, he engaged in a typical conversation with the psychologist of the adult unit. Joel discovered that he had been scheduled to lead a solution-focused group. He wondered aloud about the usefulness of engaging patients in solution-focused conversations that would be followed by problem-focused sessions with other workers. This led to a discussion about the usefulness of theory-based practice. The psychologist insisted that a practitioner "had to begin somewhere," and therefore needed a theory of the structures of what was wrong or pathological on which to base his practice. To do otherwise would be to ignore potentially "serious" conditions.

The more we engage in solution-focused practice, the more we question this stance. From its inception, the solution-focused approach emphasized an inductive orientation, asking what clients and therapists do in conversations that make a difference (Simon & Berg, 2004), tailoring conversations to clients rather than forcing clients into therapists' preconceived ideas of useful conversations.

The dictionary defines theory as "a coherent group of general propositions used as principles of explanation for a class of phenomena" (Barnhart, 1961, p. 1256). We often have heard SFBP referred to as a model or theory. Yet, as practitioners, we hold no explanations for why or how SFBP works other than the description that practice is built on what clients tell us works for them. Likewise, we have no explanations for normative behaviors and causes of psychopathology. Some therapists may find it useful to have such theories, but many equally valid ones exist, and we believe that they are not necessary in practice. In fact, when a practitioner holds to one theory, it more likely dampens possibilities than creates new ones or identifies existing potentially useful ones for the client. The therapist stays focused within that theory rather than the client's theory or context. Behaviors that exist outside the theoretical explanation are viewed as irrelevant, mere static to be ignored.

Our point is that some practitioners believe that a therapist *must* have a theory in order to practice good therapy. This is the belief with which we disagree. Although it is possible that some therapists practice good therapy from a theoretical base, we believe that inherent dangers exist and we believe that it is not *necessary* to have a theoretical base to practice good therapy.

For example, a client may state to a therapist that she is depressed 98 percent of waking hours. Theory-based practice, especially medically based, directs the practitioner to understand the depression and its ramifications. Accordingly, the therapist asks more about when the depression happens, with whom, what form it takes. The therapist may attempt to understand the etiology of the depression. From a poststructural point of view, much time and effort is spent in creating greater realities about the depression (Hoffman, 1990). Alternatively, a solution-focused practitioner's experience is that it will better serve the client to focus on the 2 percent of the time that depressive symptoms are not present:

1. When does it happen?
2. What difference does it make for the client?
3. What difference does it make for those in the client's life situation?
4. What difference would it make for the client and those who know him or her if the percentage of nondepression times were to increase?

The solution-focused therapist might then suggest to the client that she focus on the times that the 2 percent is happening and what that difference makes. Borrowing again from a poststructural orientation, such a conversation would most likely create a different reality regarding the 2 percent. Note that the SFB practitioner is not simply interested in *what* is happening in those times, but what difference it makes to the client and to others.

The authors' experience is that results of the medical language game are limited and often predictable. On the other hand, solution-building conversations increase intervention possibilities. Each intervention will have very different results depending upon the variables in the particular context; the outcomes are dynamic and uncertain. Differences that the 2 percent make for individuals are as varied as the individuals and systems involved, including such things as, "I would have more energy," "I am more pleasant to be around," and, even, "I will walk the dog." Experiences teach us that solution-focused conversations have a higher probability of constructing positive outcomes that are satisfying to both clients and others in their contexts.

It stands to reason that if we have the capacity to co-construct useful conversations, we also have the capacity to co-construct less than useful conversations. During Joel's 10-year tenure as a director of a community mental health clinic, he was amazed at the increase of referrals that took place during Mental Health Week in his local community. He learned that the local Mental Health Association would set up a display at a local shopping mall and passers-by would be encouraged to complete a "depression survey." Based on the results of the survey, people "realized" they were depressed and sought mental health services—a clear example of results being dependent upon the questions asked.

WHAT DOES THE PATIENT SAY?

A newly hired psychiatrist on the adult unit of Fairview Psychiatric Center was eager to develop a strong clinical presence. He had established a weekly case conference to review all new admissions. The psychiatrist, knowing that Joel practiced SFBP, asked him to come to a case conference to lend his "perspective."

A new female patient had been admitted the evening before, and when Joel arrived, the staff began to review the case. After discussing the precipitating events that led to her hospitalization and then a range of applicable diagnoses, the team proceeded to develop a treatment plan, including which problems were of the highest priority and what interventions and modalities were to be attempted.

Once completed, the psychiatrist turned to Joel and asked for his perspective. Joel asked, "What does the patient want to be different?" The social worker assigned to the case reiterated the patient's problems and the treatment plan the team had just agreed upon. The original question, "What does the patient want to be different?" was repeated with an identical response. Joel then asked the unit social worker, "What does the patient say that she wants to be different?" There was a moment of silence, broken when the unit director answered, "I guess nobody asked her." The difference between problem solving and solution-building is clearly illustrated. As experts, the medical team performed it's a priori–perceived function of exploring the problem, diagnosing the problem, and prescribing the treatment.

In contrast, a major principle of the solution-focused approach is that the client's stated goals for therapy are taken literally and seriously. A co-constructed therapy process begins with the client's stating what she or he wants to be different. As our colleague Harry Korman (2004) stated, "It is the client who needs to decide what changes he or she wants" (p. 3). Because we are not experts on clients' lives, we use questions as tools to help clients identify, refine, and make meaning of what they want different in their lives. If somebody else in the client's life wants something different, we work with that, too, but we make no assumptions that we must focus on pathological descriptions in order to make things better for clients.

In another example of co-constructing goals, a nineteen-year-old patient had been admitted to the adult unit at Fairview.

J: So what are you hoping will be better from being here?

P: I don't know. It wasn't my idea.

J: Okay, whose idea was it?

P: My mother. She said I was getting out of control.

J: So what would she need to see that will tell her that you are in control and it's all right for you to come home?

P: I don't know. [A pause while the therapist waits.] I guess she would hear something from the staff.

J: Of course. What do you think the staff would be saying that would tell her that it's time for you to go home?

P: I guess that I was more in control.

J: Hmmm, how would they know that?

P: I would be following the rules and going to groups and the program.

J: And when you got home, what would be going on that would tell her and maybe you as well that things are better and you probably will never have to come to a place like this again?

P: I probably would be listening to her more and helping around the house. I suppose. I would also start thinking about the future.

J: Great, what would you be thinking about the future?

P: I suppose registering for college and deciding what I want to do in life.

It often is the authors' experience that a useful conversation about therapy goals can be held once the "customer for therapy" has been identified and what needs to be different for that person is made clear. In the previous patient's case, his first and second responses clearly indicate that he was not the customer and in fact felt that he did not need to be hospitalized. An alternative conversation could have been co-constructed around his denial and resistance; the most likely result would have been greater resistance and denial. As is often the case, the therapist would have left the conversation frustrated and thinking that because of the client's steadfast refusal to accept reality, little chance existed that he would change. The client in turn would have left the conversation thinking that the therapist neither listened nor understood him.

In subsequent responses, the client expressed his understanding of what his mother wanted from him and how he needed to convince her that his behaviors had changed significantly enough for her so that he could return home. We find that it is very usual that the initial changes begin as sole responses to another's wishes. The usefulness of this position becomes evident to clients and they begin to change their behaviors, thoughts, and feelings accordingly.

As the conversation progressed, the client in our example began to discuss the future, and, specifically, his goals to attend college. Note that the therapist began by accepting the client's reality and shifted to asking not what the mother but the client himself would be thinking about the future. In response, he answered that he would be registering for college and deciding what he wants to do in life.

PSYCHIATRIC MEDICATIONS

As solution-focused therapists, we often are asked whether we harbor a negative bias against psychiatric medications. Over many years of clinical practice, clients have told us that medications have been helpful to them, and our interest always has been in how: what difference the medications make for clients and for others in the clients' lives who are important to them. Medication is one tool that clients tell us is useful. Conversations about how medications help are other useful tools; we follow the maxim of doing more of what works.

Our concern is not simply the medications themselves,[2] but the beliefs and conversations that are engendered when medications are prescribed. A doctor's prescription pad has a powerful influence in the co-constructive process. To illustrate this, consider the following composite scenario.

Jim, the mental health everyman, had had a number of recent setbacks. He had been working the same job for twenty years and had been feeling less fulfilled for quite some time. In addition, changes in management were made, and due to company downsizing, the remaining staff were forced to take on additional responsibilities. Jim now was working longer hours to complete the extra tasks and even taking work home. As a result, he was spending less time with his wife Gloria and their two children as well as on hobbies and interests that he found fulfilling.

Gloria complained about Jim's lack of availability as well as his emotional distance from her and the children. Jim had been having difficulty sleeping, and his appetite also was affected; as a result, his energy level was compromised. In the past, Jim enjoyed regular biking, but because of the job changes and increased work he was finding it harder to make room for exercise in his ever-busier schedule. He had enjoyed a weekly small-wages poker game with a few of his buddies, but had to bow out for the past two or three weeks, again because of the job changes and because he did not have enough energy to play. With all the stress, turmoil, and uncertainty, sexual activity between Jim and Gloria had been curtailed—he lacked both the energy and desire.

At the urging of his family and friends, Jim made an appointment to see a psychiatrist. Once there, he was asked the usual questions about the symptoms and family history of mental illness. Based on his responses (or, from a co-constructive point of view, based on the responses *and* the questions), the psychiatrist explained to Jim that he was suffering from major depression. The psychiatrist suggested that Jim begin a trial of antidepressant medication and, given the family history of depression and bipolar illness, explained that this most likely was a genetically based disease that had come to the fore recently because of environmental stressors. As the psychiatrist reached into his drawer, removed a prescription pad, and began to write, he explained that Jim most likely would battle depression his whole life, and that he had a disease similar to diabetes that could not be cured but could be controlled by minimizing stressors and a lifelong use of psychiatric medications.

Jim returned home and reported to his wife what the psychiatrist had said. She in turn explained to the children as best as she could that their father was having a difficult time and they needed to be extra quiet so as not to disturb him even more. One of Jim's close friends from the poker group called and asked Gloria whether Jim was planning to attend the weekly poker group. Gloria explained that Jim was diagnosed as "clinically depressed," was on medication, and needed to reduce stresses in his life. The friend expressed his understanding and stated that when Jim was ready to return to the group, he would be welcomed. In an attempt to not disturb Jim, the friend determined not to call again and told Jim's other friends about Jim's situation, who also stopped calling. Based on the psychiatrist's recommendations, Jim was granted a leave of absence from his job.

Two weeks later, Jim returned to see the psychiatrist. Jim reported that he was spending most of his time in the house watching television in his pajamas and had ceased all other activities. Jim expressed his dismay over his disability and how it made him feel hopeless and helpless. He likened his situation to a never-ending spiral downward. Concerned about Jim's emotional status, the psychiatrist referred Jim to the community inpatient mental health unit, where he was evaluated, deemed at risk for suicide, and hospitalized.

CONCLUSION

The emphasis of solution-focused conversations is on possibilities and choices. Different language games engender very different results. We have seen solution-building conversations dramatically change the direction of clients' lives. We are not opposed to psychiatric medication; we simply advocate for conversations that co-construct hope and possibilities for clients rather than conversations that predict a lifetime of doom and gloom that can become a self-fulfilling prophecy.

Wittgenstein (1958) said, "What is your aim in philosophy? To shew [*sic*] the fly the way out of the fly bottle" (p. 103). Likewise, good treatment aims to help clients find their way out of the mental health system. A conversation that centers on illness and disability constructs illness and disability. Conventional conversations within the medical model serve to keep the fly in the fly bottle, to keep therapists and clients in conversations about illness and disability. In the next chapter, we present the results of interviews with four psychiatrists who have incorporated alternative ways of thinking about and talking with their patients.

NOTES

1. Although we attempt to report the events as accurately as possible, "Fairview Hospital" is a fictitious name.
2. We also are concerned about long-term negative effects of the medicines themselves.

Chapter 7

Psychiatry Should Be a Parenthesis in People's Lives

In the previous chapter, we began a discussion regarding the medical model and its divergence from solution-focused practice. In preparation for the book, we interviewed four psychiatrists. Three are avowed solution-focused practitioners; the fourth stated that he integrates solution-focused techniques within a more traditional practice.

HARRY KORMAN

Harry Korman earned his medical degree in 1980 at Lund University in Sweden. He is a specialist in child and adolescent psychiatry. Harry works in private practice in Malmö, Sweden, with families, children, adults, and couples. He supervises and teaches Solution-Focused Brief Therapy in a number of areas within mental health and parallel fields. He worked in state-operated child and adult psychiatry for 15 years before entering private practice in 1996.

Portions of the interview were completed through e-mails in April 2004 and in May 2005. Janet Campbell also interviewed Harry in August 2001 at the Center for Solutions in New York State. Portions of this interview also are included.

Q: How do you reconcile your training as a doctor in the medical model and the ideas of SF?

HK: I don't.

Q: How does the topic of medications as a possible tool get introduced? Do you suggest it based on your idea that it might be helpful? Do you wait until the patient suggests it?

Solution-Focused Brief Practice
© 2007 by The Haworth Press, Taylor & Francis Group. All rights reserved.
doi:10.1300/5507_07

HK: The most usual situation where I do prescribe medication is that I have seen someone for maybe three, four, or five sessions, things have not improved, and I think that medication could help them move in the direction they want. I will then ask them if they have thought about medication, and I might say that it is my experience that sometimes medication can be helpful. I will try medication at that point. Sometimes it works and sometimes it doesn't. If a new client wants me to prescribe medication, I will defer any decision about this until the end of the session and if there is already some improvement (over zero on the miracle scale) I will probably not write a prescription—at least not in that session. And then there are some situations where I stop the medication.

Q: You mean that someone else has prescribed?

HK: Yes. The clients are experts on their lives. They will have ideas of how they will know that medication is useful and they will know if it has been helpful taking it or not, and thus they will also know when and if they can try without it.

Q: What kind of conversations do you have with clients about medications?

HK: "How will you notice that this medication is useful? What will be the first sign?" What do they think about medication? I think the clients' thinking about medication and ideas about medication, if they think it will be useful—that is an argument for prescribing medication. If they don't think it will be useful—that's an argument against prescribing. I think that what we do has to fit with the client's theory.

Q: Do you see medication as something that's ongoing in a person's life, or is it temporary?

HK: Oh, it's temporary until otherwise proven. For instance, with psychotic patients, I might try medication for three or maybe six months and then try without.

Q: What do you find that works in talking about medications in follow up sessions?

HK: During the time they're on the medications, talk about what they do with the possibilities that the medication creates for them. Medications don't change life; they just open up possibilities.

Q: How does the decision to stop using the medications happen? What kind of conversations seem to work?

HK: It's about trying without or finding the smallest effective dose. It's the client's job in my view. Scales are almost always useful both to make decisions and to follow up the effect of the decisions. When medication makes a big difference in someone's quality of life, the decision to try without needs serious preparation and it is a decision that needs to be taken in collaboration between the patient and the doctor.

Q: When working with, especially, "chronic" clients, do you view the use of medications as a long-term or short-term tool? Rationale for either?

HK: There is no rule here. It might be short- or long-term. You can never know—and even if it is long-term, people can stop. That goes for both antipsychotics and antidepressants.

Q: Since this is a book about brief therapy with long-term users of the mental health system, especially in the use of medications with those labeled with "chronic" diagnoses, how do you work briefly?

HK: I don't work briefly and I don't work long-term. Every session can be the last. There is no difference between so-called chronic cases and others. I have only a small clinical practice and at this time only one long-term client: schizophrenia for 15 years. I don't talk medicine with him—he has another doctor for that. Most so-called psychotic patients get better quickly with brief therapy. The last one I saw was a 32-year-old woman with a diagnosis of psychosis and drug abuse (dual diagnosis). She had "company" and she wanted to be able to turn the voices off or ignore them when she wanted and not do drugs so she could be "like everyone else." By the fifth session, she was able to do this 100 percent of the time, had moved to her own place, and was starting to see her two children who were in foster care. She stopped therapy. She was never on antipsychotics while I saw her; she had stopped that herself two years earlier because she felt "radio-guided" and got fat.

Q: How relevant is diagnosis to your practice and specifically to prescribing medications?

HK: Practically not at all. One exception is the previous case. She had a period in the middle of therapy when things became worse. She complained about hearing more voices that became threatening and she started to behave in strange ways. She told me that she wanted to stop smoking and was using an antidepressant medicine to inhibit her smoking desire. So I advised her to stop the medicine. She did and she again became able to control the voices within days. I know that this is tangential to your question. You want to know if it's useful in my practice to know whether people have schizophrenia or bipolar or other diagnosis. My answer to that question is, "practically not at all." The decision to try antidepressants, antipsychotics, or central nervous system stimulants when therapy is not successful is not very difficult.

Q: Do you discuss diagnosis with your patients? If so, how does it get introduced and how do you talk to them about diagnosis? If not, why not?

HK: I don't believe diagnosis is a useful tool, so I don't discuss it with clients. I might discuss what's helpful about "getting the right diagnosis" if the client wants to talk to me about it, but I will always add questions around what difference "getting the right diagnosis" might make in the client's life. Sometimes clients bring up diagnosis, but my experience is that most often they do this because they want to tell me that another doctor said they had X diagnosis and he or she is wrong.

Q: In what ways do SF and the "medical model" share common precepts?

HK: The pragmatics of being helpful.

Q: What kind of discussions do you have with agencies that refer someone to you—especially those that don't share the solution-focused perspective?

HK: You have to take the referral seriously. Make sure that if things don't improve immediately, you can talk to the people who are concerned. There aren't schools; there are people in schools who are concerned, caring, and worried. What is it that they need to see happen as a result of what I do? What will be signs for them that therapy is being useful?

Q: So, this is the conversation that you have with them.

HK: Yes. They are the ones that care about what happens. They are the judges of if what I do is useful or not. My business is to do what I do; their job is to evaluate the effect of it. Their business is not to tell me what to do.

Q: So how do you respond to someone who says, "You need to see this person once a week," "This child needs intense therapy," or, "This child has bipolar disorder"?

HK: "Okay, so let's say I see him once a week, how will you see it's helpful to him?"

Q: "Well, I think it will take a long time for things to happen."

HK: "Sure, sure. So what will be the first sign that the work I'm doing is useful?"

Q: "He would start off the day without being agitated."

HK: "Wouldn't be agitated; that would be the first sign."

Q: "Yes."

HK: "So, what would be the first sign that this was starting to happen—not being agitated?"

Q: "He would be able to come in and settle down, be able to hear instructions."

HK: "Hear instructions, settle down; what would be the very first, small sign that this was happening?"

Q: Thanks, that was helpful. Sometimes I find that when I ask similar questions, the referring person seems to be annoyed. I guess they're not used to being asked these kinds of questions.

HK: If they start getting irritated at my questions, I will explain that it is very important for me to know. They are the only ones that can tell me. I think the essence of solution-focused therapy is what people want.

Q: In a general way, how do you see your role as a psychiatrist?

HK: I think psychiatry should be a parenthesis in people's lives, not the contrary. Sometimes, psychiatry acts as if life is a parenthesis in people's psychiatry. I shouldn't be the most important person in people's lives. We should do as little as possible.

ALASDAIR MACDONALD

Alasdair Macdonald earned his medical degree at the University of Glasgow, Glasgow, Scotland, and completed postgraduate training at the University of Dundee Medical School in Dundee, Scotland. He has been a consulting psychiatrist in the British National Health Service for 25 years. He has experience in acute general psychiatry, psychiatric intensive care units, and psychotherapy. His psychotherapy training includes psychodynamic, group, and systemic approaches. Alasdair is registered as a family therapist and supervisor with the United Kingdom Council for Psychotherapy. He has been the medical director of two trusts and the project director of the Mental Health Institute, St. Martin's College at Carlisleand and Lancaster for the past 16 years, his major focus has been teaching and training in Solution-Focused Brief Therapy. He has taught and presented in the UK, Europe, Australia, and the United States and has special experience in the application of SFBT ideas within mental health settings and with offenders. Currently, his main research interest is in the study of process and outcomes in SFBT.

Q: How do you reconcile your training in the medical model and the ideas of SF?

AM: The medical model is one way of addressing problems; SFBT is usually a better way and will meet less resistance from the client because it is collaborative.

Q: How do you reconcile your perceived role as the "medical expert" and the SF orientation toward the client as expert?

AM: I listen to the client but remain alert for patterns which may signify illness (physical or mental) or goals which could be addressed by a medical intervention as one option.

Q: How does the topic of medications as a possible tool, get introduced? Do you suggest it based on your idea that it might be helpful? Do you wait until the patient suggests it?

AM: Some ask for medication or I may suggest it.

Q: Whether initiated by you or the patient, how do you introduce the topic of medication?

AM: For involuntary patients I might say, "Medication may be helpful to you in achieving your goal. We will find it hard to work with you if you do not accept medication." For voluntary clients, I might say, "I have seen others with similar stories who have benefited from medication." I will then suggest they try a medication as an experiment for a specified period of time. I find this helpful for negotiation.

Q: What do you find that works in talking about medications in follow-up sessions?

AM: After, "What's better?" I ask, "Did you take the medication? Did it help?"

Q: How does the decision to stop using the medications happen?

AM: Sometimes I advise that a change of medication is advisable; sometimes they or I will say that they can try without it now, and then we negotiate.

Q: What kind of conversations seem to work?

AM: All changes to medications should be framed as "slowly," with advice on when or whether to slow or reverse the changes.

Q: I've found in talking to clients who are taking medications that they often "blame" the medications for improvements. What have you found useful in shifting the agency of positive change?

AM: "You have done a lot yourself, although the medications may also have helped. You have been able to do these things in the past without taking medications."

Q: Since this is a book about brief therapy with long-term users of the mental health system, especially in the use of medications with those labeled with "chronic" diagnoses, how do you work briefly?

AM: Clients usually have specific problems when they attend. They admit to them or these are identified by someone else, for example, a relative or professional. The client and I work with that using SFBT. Afterward, I will either discharge the client or reorient the therapy to "support" once the problem is managed adequately. The medication should be maintained at the lowest effective dose, with increases when the situation requires it. This reduces side effects and increases compliance.

Q: How relevant is diagnosis to your practice and specifically to prescribing medications?

AM: Identified symptoms may respond to specific drugs; major diagnostic categories are less reliable as predictors of response. Antidepressants reduce the symptoms of formal depression until the episode is past. They sometimes help the mood in depressive spectrum disorders. Antipsychotics improve mental functioning and behavior control in those with a major psychosis, thus assisting psychological and psychosocial interventions. Antipsychotics impair mental function in those who do not have psychosis. Otherwise, I prescribe for symptoms rather than for diagnosis.

Q: Do you discuss diagnosis with your patients? If so, how does it get introduced and how do you talk to them about diagnosis? If not, why not?

AM: In major psychosis and bipolar disorder, I will tell the patient if they ask or if it is necessary to their forward planning (for example, a court order specifying "schizophrenia" is going to make a difference for the patient). Otherwise, I use whatever name the patient wants to call the problem. If they ask what ICD-10 or DSM-IV will call it, then I tell them. You can use this conversation to discuss prognosis and therefore likely exceptions with them. The hospital paperwork usually requires an official diagnostic classification, but this has little bearing on my conversation with the patient.

Q: When working with clients, especially with "chronic" clients, do you view the use of medications as a long-term or short-term tool? Rationale for either?

AM: Long-term medication is needed for a number of clients with major psychosis or resistant depression. Long-term studies on major psychosis have shown that by middle age, many patients require little or no medication. For most other long-term problems, the need for medication varies from time to time.

Q: What do the medical model and SFBT have in common?

AM: The medical model is essentially a pattern-recognition exercise. A music buff can hear a few bars, recognize the piece, and predict the whole pattern, maybe for hours at a time. A gardener can see an anonymous green shoot in their garden, and say, "In two weeks that will be a [blank] plant and it will need some time if it is going to be the right shape." In medicine you do this by listening to clients, looking for exceptions (although I have never heard it called that), and recognizing that problems and solutions may appear different. (Ambrose Bierce suggested that tablets were like throwing stones in one neighborhood to kill a dog in another part of town). But medicine has an expert knowledge mindset; it is based on action by the medical authority, and for good reasons it is linked to the fastest possible change/repair. These qualities seem to me different from SF thinking.

RALPH DAHLE

Ralph Dahle was interviewed in May 2004 and July 2005. Dahle lives in close proximity to the interviewer, and this allowed for a more extensive conversation. He received his medical degree in 1981 at the College of Osteopathic Medicine, at Des Moines University in Des Moines, Iowa, and received his board certification in psychiatry in 1985. Dr. Dahle is in private practice in Harrisburg, Pennsylvania, and has consulted at both state and general hospitals. Dahle replied in writing to an initial set of questions sent by the interviewer prior to the actual face-to-face conversation.

Q: How do you reconcile your training as a doctor in the medical model and the ideas of SF?

RD: I sometimes apply the medical model and sometimes SF. They are not exclusionary; applying both is what I do most.

Q: Give me an example of how you do that.

RD: I'll use a worst-case scenario: a schizophrenic patient—let's say paranoid. He comes in reporting that he's doing "normal" things like taking a trip to Chicago, which required getting on the plane and being with people. He did it and I supported his success. He's still paranoid, but that's all right. The medical model would be the medication but an SF model would be supporting his efforts to do things on his own that involve counter-stances to his condition.[1] He was able to go out and be out in a strange city. I think that worked against his normal stance of being isolated and staying home.

Q: Taking that example, when he returns from Chicago, what kind of conversation do you have with him at that point?

RD: I stay with what was fun, what he enjoyed, what he was able to do. He likes to drift into what is miserable in life; I try to keep him on what is uplifting. What worked about the trip?

Q: What kind of conversation did you have before he went?

RD: We didn't. We talked before about what is better for him: getting out of the house. We talked about what wasn't so useful for him: staying in this isolated position. One way that people do that is taking a trip. Then he went. We didn't plan the event.

Q: Did that idea exist before your conversation?

RD: No—not that I was aware of.

Q: So, your conversation may have co-constructed that reality?

RD: Yes, if I understand the concept of "co-construction" correctly.

Q: In conventional psychoanalysis, he would probably be repri-
manded because you're not supposed to do anything without consulting with the psychoanalyst to make sure you're not "acting
out." If you consider the conversation you had with him as being
more oriented to an SF approach versus the medical model, which
tends to focus more on diagnosis and symptom management, how
do you decide which focus you're going to take?

RD: I suppose when the symptoms become so relevant that they interfere with other things. So, if he were getting so psychotic and hearing voices, not going anywhere, I would have to be a little firmer,
"This is your condition; this is what we need to do. Are you willing
to do it?" I would also intervene if the symptoms interfere with the
conversation with me. I have a woman who stopped her medications. She is crumbling. It interferes in the relationship with me.
She starts screaming for no reason. At that point, I might suggest
that she get back on her medication. Explain how they were helpful—they're part of the solution. I know it's her choice, but I
strongly recommend it. I take SF to mean that the person has the
capacity to do what is corrective. On some level, the medical
model includes the same perspective.

Q: Say more about that. What do you mean? I know I have the tendency to highlight the differences. I'm interested in: What are the
similarities?

RD: The medical model assumes that the body has a corrective response. Harry Korman [1997] says in his article that most illnesses
get cured in their own anyway. I think the medical model incorpo-
rates a self-correcting system. The antibiotic only helps the im-
mune system—it doesn't replace it. We can do surgery to remove a
tumor because the body will heal that injury but might not heal the
injury of the tumor. We know the body has the capacity to heal itself. On the body level, it's a solution-focused model.

Q: What happened philosophically in the practice in psychotherapy,
where the practitioner has become the expert on the person?

RD: I was trained as a doctor of osteopathy; I think the approach is
much more holistic. I also think part of the problem is an East

Coast arrogance that is not present in the Midwest. I think psychiatrists there are more open to trying something different and seeing if it works. I think it's a regional difference; I was trained in the Midwest. I think we don't know that we've become arrogant. I think we become controlling because we feel so out of control. We get overwhelmed with the inherent powerlessness we have sometimes.

Q: Among your colleagues, is there a general assumption that we will get to the point in psychiatry where we can treat as an immunologist treats?

RD: Yes, I think that's the *Zeitgeist.* Right now the hope is genetics. I suppose then it's easy to go from there to acting as if it's already true. Yes, that's the dilemma.

Q: In your original responses to me, you said, "When I'm feeling pessimistic, I think all we can do is palliative. At other times, I firmly believe we can change our mind." Regarding the latter, what do you think when you change your mind?

RD: I fall back on my own experiences of my own life. When I change the way I think, I feel differently. So I know I can change my mind. I'm more positive about patients; I'm more optimistic. I don't bring my pessimism into the office. I stay to what helps and what's positive in their lives. I tell my clients that not only can they change their minds, but also they can change their brains. We're starting to see that this is true in research. Every conversation goes down a different neural pathway. That's what I tell patients. "The more you stay with the negative, the more you pave that negative street."

Q: We can map where activity is active in the brain. This kind of research has demonstrated that psychotherapy can likely change the brain. If, as you said, a positive conversation with a therapist will have a concomitant positive effect on the brain, wouldn't it likely be true that any conversation with anyone that comes into a client's life has a potential for creating changes?

RD: Yes.

Q: Why then are conventional therapies geared more to therapist and client?

RD: We've been geared to look at the negative, to spend time looking at what's wrong. The longer I practice, the more I'm convinced that this is mistaken. For example, this guy comes in and tells me how miserable he feels and asks me how often I feel on top of the world. I tell him every day. He replies that he feels that way once every six months and he says he doesn't feel engaged with people. I ask him how he feels here with me. He replies he feels pretty good because we always connect. He recognizes that there's an exception. We're not focusing on how miserable he is but the exception, which is happening in the office with me.

Q: Wouldn't it also be so, wouldn't the opposite have an effect as well, that paving the negative road can have a negative effect on brain chemistry?

RD: That's my concern. Some psychotherapy actually fosters disease. If you're talking all negatively for an hour, and we assume that everything we do goes through our brains, maybe that's a side effect of psychotherapy. I think that's what the goal will be in the future, to see how conversations affect brain chemistry; maybe we won't need chemicals in the future. Maybe we can do it experientially and that will lead to a stronger individual.

Q: Regarding being the medical expert, you said, "That's easy, I don't buy into it. I do have knowledge that the client doesn't have: pharmacology, physiology. When I work, I stress collaboration as the client is the expert when it comes to their responses to interventions." How do you stress that collaborative relationship with the client?

RD: I say to a person, "You have a depression that maybe medicines will help. It's up to you." I tell them that I don't have the power to make them take it; it's their choice. The message is, "We have to do this together." I also tell them that they need to let me know how the medication is working.

Q: What about the use of medication? What kind of conversations do you have about medications?

RD: I ask them about their goals: "How will you know that I'm helping you. What do you want from me?"

Q: When you finally conclude that meds would be helpful, how do you address that?

RD: You have someone saying, "I'm not the same as I used to be; I'm not having as much fun. My friends notice I'm not going out as much as I used to, that I'm not as happy as I used to be. They're asking what's wrong with me. I can't get out of bed in the morning. Everything is a chore." I say, "Sounds like you could use some help with that. These medications could help." I discuss the costs: side effects.

Q: You said, the hard part is suggesting *not* using the medication? What works?

RD: Being a physician, most of my patients are seeing another practitioner for the psychotherapy, so I don't do the psychological treatment. And most of those folks are not doing SF treatment. I am sort of stuck in this system that's part of the problem. I try to finagle my way out of it as best as I can by putting it all back on the person.

Q: How do you do that?

RD: I might tell them something like, "I'll work with you; medications might be helpful." For some patients, I think medicines are baloney; they're not going to help. Usually they come in after being on everything in the book. I might say, "Here are some other options, but from my experience what you have sounds like medicines are not for you. You just don't have what we can treat with medicines. Doesn't mean you can't be treated; it just means you can't be treated with medications." I have to put the caveat in there that I can be wrong. Sometimes I've been surprised. It could be the placebo effect, or you moved into another brain pattern, which is what the placebo effect is: it's hope. "It you want to try the medicine, here's what you haven't been on and we can try."

Q: Do you ever remember a case that a patient took that as a positive thing?

RD: Oh, yeah, there are people who don't want to be on medicine.

Q: When you say to them, "I don't think this is going to be useful for you," do some people say, "Gee, maybe I can handle this on my own"?

RD: No, I think that's because the therapists that they're working with are not solution-focused. They're not having that kind of conversation. What I in essence say to them is, "You have done it on your own, you're sitting here talking to me, you've done okay in spite of all this. You've never acted on suicide—here are the danger signals—you haven't endangered yourself, you haven't lost your job, you're not crazy, you're not hearing voices. Those are the danger signals. If you have those, I would recommend medicine a little more strongly. I'm still not saying you have to be on them; I'm not going to follow you home, and I can't make you take it."

Q: In recent years, there have been more and more commercials on television: social anxiety, take this medication, ask your doctor. Has that changed your practice?

RD: Some, not much. Once in awhile, someone will come in and say they saw something about Paxil and they're on Zoloft. Or these people who come in with PTSD and say these medicines work and I say I haven't seen them work. That's the kind of person I say, "I don't think what you have is responsive to medicines."

Q: You said collaboration is the key with the client being the expert in terms of response. What do you mean, "Collaboration is the key?"

RD: I don't know what the medicine is going to do to them. I need them to tell me. I want to know what's different on the medications, either positive or negative effects.

Q: If a client comes to you and says, "I'm okay, I don't think I need the medicine anymore," what kind of conversation do you have then?

RD: Here is where diagnosis is important to me. Let's say the person had a history of going through this before, what are the warning signals? I think I'm probably more in the medical model here than SF. I would say, "Fine. Let's work together on this." I try to keep it collaborative. It's a choice. I think it's fair to express the risk increases directly to the number of episodes.

Q: Is there an assumption that you make if possible: It's better not to use meds than use meds?

RD: The answer is yes, but I think it's a bias. It's probably a general cultural bias. It's better not to use medication if you can. I'm not sure it's a beneficial bias, but I do think I have that.

Q: You said, "Medication along with other changes are more likely to be effective; that is, doing the things that work if they are not destructive to the process are to be continued, and if reasonable, increased." How do you get the client to see that?

RD: With great difficulty.

Q: In what cases have you been successful?

RD: It's not my success, it's the patient's ability to hear it and accept it. I bring it up. I'll give you an example. I have a patient that I would describe as an anxious guy, but who is fairly successful. I asked him, "Anxiety is predicting the future. Can you do that?" He responds, "No." We tried some medicines, they really didn't do much. I took him off. He came back and said I gave him good advice. He said, "I catch myself when I'm getting ahead of myself." He went on about how beneficial the advice has been. He looked at me and said, "Wintertime is coming. And that affects my business." So, I said to him, "So, when's the last time you starved?" You could see the light go off. He caught it. He was able to do it.

Q: You said, "[You] don't work briefly; this is chronic care. That doesn't mean there isn't much that can't be done in a brief therapy model. Treatment is multifaceted, and not exclusionary." Can you say more about that?

RD: I have a lot of people I see once a year for medication. I see them once a year because they and I assume it's best they stay on the medication. They do a lot of things on their own. For example, they're exercising now when they weren't before. They're applying what we've talked about. Recently I got a letter from a woman who is legally blind. Her physician added that she has a great attitude. She wrote, "My great attitude is because of you." We talked about things like not predicting disasters in the future. I don't have a theory about that—she was able to do it. She's on low-level medication. She's "chronic" in the sense that she's connected to me once a year in a miniscule way—and maybe chronic in the sense that she's connected to me intellectually and internally because I told her, "I don't have to worry about that." She has that perception of me. She's doing well in life, and that was a brief intervention.

Q: I find a lot of the time that people attribute changes to the medications. To me that's problematic—I want them to take ownership of what's better. I'm neutral about the prescribing of medication because I think for clients, what works, works. What's your sense of that?

RD: I give them the credit for taking the medication. The medicine can't do anything without the patient. They are very much involved in their treatment. These are potent medications—we know they do something to the brain. They are taking them and so they are doing something to help themselves. I wouldn't argue with them because it's working.

Q: Regarding diagnosis, you said, "Possibly diagnosis could be done without when working with the client and just use their goals as the criteria for improvement, which is what I try to do." How do you do that?

RD: I ask them how they will know that I'm helping them. They are often befuddled by it. When you get from them their criteria of what they want to be different, you can then put a label on it. That's what a diagnosis is—the negative of the goal.

Q: You said, "Diagnoses is not an absolute necessity for prescribing medications, using the goals of the patient can be used. The goals often fit diagnostic criteria." What meaning does the client take from a diagnosis?

RD: They don't tell me. I just give a number. It might have more serious impact than I know. Half the time, they're coming from someone else with a diagnosis, and I ask what the other therapist is calling them.

SOPHIE DURIEZ

Dr. Duriez says of herself:

> When I began my career as a psychiatrist and therapist in France and continued in Germany, I had no idea I would become one of the very few solution-focused psychiatrists in the United States. I am board certified in general psychiatry and have practiced in community clinics. As a child psychiatrist, I will soon be working at the Los Angeles juvenile hall and also have a private practice in Los Angeles. My background training as a therapist is in family systems and constructivist approaches. I first did training in family therapy in Europe with the Italians (Gianfranco Cecchin, Maurizio Andolfi, etc.) during the 1980s. I am still a member of the European Family Therapy Association. I also trained at the Mental Research Institute (MRI) in Palo Alto, California in 1990. With MRI, I founded the Association for Brief Therapy Development in Paris in 1991 and organized three international conferences: one in Palo Alto and two in France with MRI. In 1993, I moved to Heidelberg and worked at the Heidelberg Systemic Institute with Fritz Simon. While in Heidelberg, I first met Steve de Shazer during a congress on constructivism in 1991. This encounter was fun, stimulated my curiosity in the solution-focused approach, and I started reading solution-focused literature.

In 1998, I moved to Los Angeles. I contacted Drs. Jennifer Andrews and David Clark, and they have allowed me to stay in contact with the postmodern therapy community. Thanks to them, I have been able to be a member of the Solution-Focused Brief Therapy Association (SFBTA) since it's creation in 2003. I first met Insoo Kim Berg in 2003 at the first SFBTA conference organized by Jennifer in Loma Linda, California. I've come to admire Insoo Kim Berg's spirit, courage, remarkable talent, and creativity in therapy. I am honored to have had her support and interest in what I am doing.

I have published a few articles in French and in English. I love constructivism—especially applied constructivism or the practice of constructivism. I knew Heinz von Foerster very well and presented with him and Ernst von Glasersfeld in European conferences during the 1990s. In my experience, the solution-focused approach was a natural evolution of the MRI model and constructivist approach. While I haven't been formally trained in SF, I find it marvelously matches my therapeutic perspective. I have started practicing SF during my U.S. psychiatric training and as a community psychiatrist. Since 2005, I presented workshops in solution-focused conferences both in the United States and in Europe based on my experience of integrating the SF approach within the conventional medical model of mental health care. I am currently writing a brief SF approach guide for people working within the psychiatric field.

Q: How do you reconcile your training in the medical model and the ideas of solution focus?

SD: In my case, my training in the medical model has never been an obstacle to the ideas of the solution-focused approach. I chose to specialize in psychiatry after I read *Change* by Watzlawick, Weakland, and Fisch [1974] more than twenty years ago. At that time, I was a medical student in France, ready to give up medicine for an acting career. I was also a student in a dramatic art school. The book was a revelation; instead of leaving medical school to become an actor, I found it more exciting to train for the role of a "real" psychiatrist who could perform "live" with the people acting as clients. Therefore, I play the role without subscribing to the medical biological model. Years later, solution-focused ideas came naturally to me as being a genius evolution of the MRI model. Interestingly, there are common points between the biomedical model and the solution-focused approach. Both of them are present- and future-oriented, and subscribe to a similar philosophy: "Problem talking," as well as knowing more about the history of the problem, aren't necessary to solve problems, and problems can be overcome within a brief period of time. Nevertheless, the medical model has a linear problem, deficit-oriented perspective, which makes the solution-focused approach radically different from it.

Q: How do you reconcile your perceived role as the "medical expert" and the solution-focused orientation toward the client as expert?

SD: I think I partly answered this question. My perceived role as the "medical expert" is up to me. If I start believing in my medical expertise, I lose the whole process of the solution-focused orientation and remain a conventional, deficit-based or problem-oriented psychiatrist. A client's expertise is so much more interesting than the medical expertise—that's probably the reason why I never subscribed to the belief of being a medical expert of people's problems.

Q: How does the topic of medications as a possible tool get introduced? Do you suggest it based on your idea that it might be helpful? Do you wait until the patient suggests it? Other alternatives that might happen?

SD: It all depends on the context. As much as possible, it is preferable to first ask the patient what he or she thinks about medications as one way among others to reach his or her goal. The best situation is when the patient comes to see you "fresh," meaning without medications and expectation for an already made diagnosis. Nowadays, when someone goes to see a psychiatrist, most of the time it is with the expectation to be prescribed medications. In the same way, patients are referred to me from another MD, family member, therapist, family practitioner, school counselor, etc. for medication prescription. Somehow, if you don't prescribe medications, you are not doing your job as a psychiatrist. So, it is an interesting challenge to deal with the pressure to prescribe. It is always possible to ask the miracle question and then move on to scaling. Medication prescription can be done in a solution-focused spirit. For instance, it is useful to ask what the patient will do (or has done) to help the medication work. It is also useful to redefine medications as being only a little part of the path to the solution. The biomedical model considers pharmacotherapy as being the solution per se; that's where solution-focused reframing is needed.

Q: Whether initiated by you or the patient, how do you introduce the topic of medication?

SD: When you are a psychiatrist in the United States, the topic of medication is implicit as soon as you see a patient. Sometimes, psychiatrists are called, "psychopharmacologists." The best way to deal with this implicit situation is to make it explicit. First, let the patient speak. Sometimes, patients are very educated about DSM-IV diagnosis and psychiatric treatment. Let's say that a patient states that he has a bipolar disorder and that he is taking this and that medication. He would like to have your opinion about his treatment. How is he doing right now: that's what I would ask. If he says, "Fine, I am stable," it is useful to ask what happened for him to get diagnosed with a bipolar disorder, what is his definition of bipolar disorder, how did it manifest, and what action he took to become stable. *Stable* is a vague term; what is the patient's definition of "stable"? How does he describe his "stable" state? It is always possible to compliment the patient, inquire how he helped the medication to work for him, and also ask him the miracle question. In this example, I would certainly keep the medication the way it has been prescribed. If it is working for the patient, I don't fix it. On the other hand, if the patient complains of side effects and other problems, I would ask what he thinks about medications and work with him from his position. In general, patients open up easily if they feel that what they say is seriously taken into consideration.

If a patient is not taking medications and comes to see you for something called "panic attacks," very often he expects to be helped by medication. The pitfall to avoid in such cases is what I call the "freezing" of a situation that becomes labeled with a diagnosis and mechanically fixed by medications. The way you engage with the patient will determine the course of the follow-up. Solution-focused ideas are very helpful to keep the therapeutic process dynamic. Exception questions and compliments are very effective. I remember a patient who found it very helpful to carry pills in his pocket for a while without necessarily taking them. The idea that he had immediate access to instant relief was a powerful help. I think that psychiatrists don't use solution-focused ideas because they don't know the approach. When I speak with my colleagues, most often they are very interested and receptive to solution-focused ideas.

Q: What do you find that works in talking about medications in follow-up sessions?

SD: I found that what works is to ask the patient a percentage question. Let's say that she feels improved. What is the percent of the improvement due to medications, and what percent is due to actions taken by the patient? In community clinics, follow up medication management monthly sessions last fifteen minutes. In private practice, it's more often twenty minutes. Even if this is a short time, it is very possible to apply solution-focused ideas. You base your intervention from a strength-based approach instead of a deficit-based approach. Medication may be reframed as a supporting agent for a patient's progress toward her goal. With the percentage question, it is possible to ask how the patient thinks she could increase the percentage of her action. This can be done together with scaling.

Q: How does the decision to stop using the medications happen? What kind of conversations seem to work?

SD: The decision to stop medication should happen naturally as a gentle, gradually decreasing process while encouraging and supporting the client's continuous action for his ongoing well-being and solution finding. Unfortunately, what happens most of the time is that clients as well as psychiatrists are afraid of stopping medications. Traditionally, the patient is viewed as somebody who needs to follow the directions of a medical expert in order to compensate for his biological pathology. It is a very common belief in psychiatry that some mental conditions necessitate medications for life, that is, bipolar disorder, schizophrenia, etc. From the biomedical standpoint, especially in those cases of "lifetime" conditions, the client's responsibility to take action to improve and modify her behavior doesn't exist. The problem presented by the patient is interpreted and categorized as a pathological process due to the lack or surplus of some biochemical neurotransmitter. Thus, the patient is the passive recipient of psychotropic medication correcting her chemical imbalance.

As Janet Bavelas and others [Bavelas, McGee, Phillips, & Routledge, 2000] show in their "Microanalysis of Communication in Psychotherapy" [article], medication becomes the focus rather than the person taking it. When a psychiatrist talks to a patient, it is common for him to say that a certain medication "works well" or "does a good job," etc. Following the biomedical model, the medication is the subject and the patient the object. Psychiatrists often equate chronic medical conditions (e.g., diabetes) to mental conditions. Imagine if you remove the daily insulin treatment from a diabetic person, you kill that person. So, to touch the medication treatment of a chronic user of mental health services may be considered not only a very risky business but medical malpractice as well. In this context, it is difficult to imagine how a person with a label of "chronic condition" can stop taking medications. Moreover, for a patient labeled with chronicity, taking medications and going to traditional therapy most often becomes like a job for which the patient may receive a disability income. As I don't subscribe to the belief of chronic mental illness, when I meet with a person labeled with a chronic mental condition, I engage in a conversation focusing on what works right now, what has been working for this person, and how this person manages to keep doing what is working for her. If the person is a great complainer, completely filled with negativity, I will acknowledge her complaints and possibly compliment her for being such a great complainer and move on with solution-building. The miracle question is a very useful tool to completely reverse the patient's perspective one hundred and eighty degrees around and make it possible for her to consider discontinuing medication. To gently give responsibility back to the person and to support her sustained efforts to make a better life for herself is the goal to be achieved when beginning the process of discontinuing the medication.

Q: I've found in talking to clients who are taking meds that they often "blame" the medications for improvements. What have you found useful in shifting the agency of positive change?

SD: You point exactly to the problem created by medication intake within a linear medical model! Sometimes, to ask whether the positive change is due to his initiative or to medication can be very surprising for clients. A client once told me, "I never thought I could do something good!" Clients have great trouble recognizing their positive changes as being due to themselves. How could they do differently when they have been told that they have a chemical imbalance and that the medication compensates for the imbalance? Then, they've been told that the possibility of relapse is always present. If a client is convinced that his brain is inadequate, it's difficult for him to imagine something different. When the brain is blamed for being the problem, the brain's natural response is to become the problem—that maintains the problem. Often, as I have mentioned previously, the antiproblem medication is personified and thus receives all the praises and compliments when the patient feels his situation has improved.

I find it useful to shift the agency of positive change to help the client alter his perspective of his situation. For example, I saw a patient while covering for her regular psychiatrist. She had a twenty-year history of anxiety and was coming for her monthly medication prescription. I asked her the miracle question. After having answered and positioned herself on the scale, she looked at me and said, "I can't believe it. For twenty years, I feel like I have been knocking at a closed door and I just realized now that there was a whole landscape behind me. I just needed to turn around." This comment is one of the best descriptions I have ever heard about the extraordinary effects of the miracle question.

Q: Since this is a book about brief therapy with long-term users of the mental health system, especially in the use of medications with those labeled with "chronic" diagnoses, how do you work briefly?

SD: Long-term psychiatric clients have often completely adopted the idea they are nothing but failures. Somehow, they have mastered a degree in personal and social failure. They are ostracized from their families, from their work environment, and often they are homeless. Medication is the only contact they have with other people at their local mental health clinic. They often indulge in street drugs, which has the double advantage of immediate gratification while pursuing their self-destruction and belonging to a street social network. The person within this context maintains her position as an expert in life failure. Insoo Kim Berg says, "you need to be slow to go fast." If you want to work briefly with long-term mental health clients, you need to take your time. Asking unusual questions and, specifically, the miracle question works very well with these clients. Long-term users labeled with "chronic" diagnoses know exactly what to expect from traditional mental health providers: the same linear, paternalistic, well-intentioned medical questions, over and over. So, if you throw unexpected questions, somehow it wakes the client up to new possibilities. In this, the solution-focused presupposition radically differs from the traditional one. The medical presupposition, which is pathological and deficit-based, tends to reify "chronic" clients as if they are broken human machines. Solution focus speaks to strengths and competencies. To quote Milton Erickson, "The patient knows the solution to his problem. Only he doesn't know that he knows." The therapist is there only to help the patient reconnect with his own strengths, competencies, and expertise. The "chronic" client's expertise can be transferred from failure and self-destruction to success and self-care. I have seen some "chronic" clients move from the street and jail back to home and family.

Q: How relevant is diagnosis to your practice and specifically to prescribing medications?

SD: Diagnosis brings the whole issue of the medical model used in psychiatry. In medicine and surgery, diagnosis is crucial in order to prescribe the correct treatment. While diagnosis is relevant to medicine and surgery, it is less so when applied to psychiatry. Diagnosis in psychiatry is a label, which presumes the existence of underlying brain pathology—a chemical imbalance. It looks scientific, but so far the famous chemical imbalance is only a hypothesis and not a demonstrated fact. For sure, our brain chemistry is always changing. At any given moment, we may experience many chemical changes as our state of mind and emotions constantly vary and react to our environment. If I receive good news, my brain makes me happy but if I learn bad news, it makes me sad. When it comes to psychiatric practice, the therapeutic effects start together with the diagnostic process. I want to create a surprising chemical imbalance, or, in other words, I aim to induce a corrective emotional thought through a conversation with the client. Instead of looking for symptoms, I will first evaluate the client's position vis-à-vis his problem. Is he a therapy customer or is he a visitor sent by his spouse, the judge, or somebody else? Who is talking to me? Therefore, the relevance of diagnosis to my practice is variable because it depends on the context in which the client presents himself.

Diagnosis is an important factor to take under consideration when the client already carries a "lifetime" diagnosis when he comes to see me. If it is the case, how does the client position himself vis-à-vis his diagnosis? This is helpful to explore in order to orient the conversation as soon as possible to what is working well for the client. In general, when you talk to people about what they do well, they are surprised and they appreciate it. That's where I get the emotional corrective thought I am looking for. Some clients have a collection of diagnoses and they identify themselves as their collection. A client might tell me, "I have ADHD, bipolar disorder, PTSD, social phobia, and panic attacks. I'm also a borderline and therefore I need this or that medication." I will compliment the client on having so many diagnoses and yet keeping himself together. Then I would ask how he manages to do that despite all of his diagnoses.

What I find also useful is to identify what are the client's expectations from me. If the expectation is medication prescription, I won't oppose the request, but I will ask questions—unexpected questions like the miracle question, scaling, or other stimulating solution-focused questions. Often, the diagnosis itself is the only problem. For instance, it is unfortunately very common for some clients who are going through a particularly difficult time to get quickly diagnosed with a chronic diagnosis. This may happen if one of their parents is already diagnosed with an "inheritable mental illness" (e.g., bipolar disorder). They might be preventively prescribed a mood stabilizer in order to hinder further development of their own possible inherited bipolar disorder.

When I meet a client in this context, I try to translate the psychiatric diagnosis into a description of the problem in ordinary simple terms. I don't let myself get intimidated by an already made diagnosis. When someone comes without a previous diagnosis, I evaluate the client's situation with the client and will assess on one hand what is the problem and on the other what are the client's specific resources, strengths, and competencies. Then I will ask the miracle and scaling questions. It also helps to explore exceptions to the problem and what has been working in the past. This helps the client figure how he can move towards his miracle. I am solution-focused and client-centered. At the time of establishing concrete solution steps, I will ask the client whether she might consider medications and then prescribe if the client believes that it would be useful to help her accomplish her path toward a solution. I will orient the conversation to let the client actively decide how she will make the medication work for her.

Q: Do you discuss diagnosis with your patients? If so, how does it get introduced and how do you talk to them about diagnosis? If not, why not?

SD: Yes, I think it is very important to discuss diagnosis, or better to discuss the idea of diagnosis with my patients. It is always interesting to get an idea of what patients think about a label. Diagnoses are now part of mainstream vocabulary, and some of them are very popular, like bipolar or ADHD. Those labels reinforce the common idea that there is something permanently wrong in their brains. Once, I had a patient who believed he had a bipolar disorder. He had been told some years ago that this was his condition. He had been given medications for years and didn't think that psychotherapy was an option for him. He was resigned to the idea that he not only had a chronic condition but that this condition was highly inheritable and therefore he didn't want to have children.

When finally he made a monitored trial of gradually discontinuing his meds, he realized he could live without his meds. The diagnosis was dropped together with the meds. However, for him to give up the idea that he was a chronic psychiatric case was not so easy. He had to take responsibility for his thoughts and behavior from now on, and this was very challenging.

His long distance girlfriend (herself diagnosed and medically treated for chronic depression) was very upset with this new change of status. He got into an argument with her about it and she attributed his disagreement with her to his "untreated condition." She wanted him to have a second opinion, otherwise she would leave him. He had had more than a second opinion as I had presented his case (with him coming for an interview) to the entire staff of the teaching psychiatry university department. After discussion, the staff agreed on a diagnosis of generalized anxiety disorder, history of alcohol abuse, and dependent personality traits—adios, bipolar disorder. He gave the girlfriend the case conference written presentation but that was not enough for her. I invited her to come with him for a session, but she refused, and finally she dropped him.

His change of label was a revealing experience, allowing him to experience his style of relating to people. This was a tremendous challenge for him, but he handled it. Chronic labels take away responsibility from people, and usually they establish their lifestyle based on those disabling labels. Also, those labels may become essential for a source of income when "chronic patients" apply for disability income.

The impact of diagnosis is powerful on multiple levels: within the individual, the family, the socioeconomic, and the political systems. Therefore, I believe that to avoid discussing labels and their implications with patients is a mistake. Generally, to introduce the topic of diagnosis, after having listened to the complaint, I ask the patient if a physician, a therapist, or a family member had ever given her or him a diagnosis. If not, has [she or] he ever thought of how her or his problem could be labeled and how the exceptions to the problem could be labeled too. I believe it is very important to ask questions about the exceptions to the problems as soon as possible, as well as what has worked in the past, and then the resources, skills, and strengths of the person. I like to make two lists: the list of "what's going wrong" (that which brought the person in for the consultation) and the list of "what's going well." The second list is used as a basis to overcome the problems of list one.

Q: When working with clients, especially "chronic" clients, do you view the use of medications as a long-term or short-term tool? Rationale for either?

SD: When working with "chronic clients," I generally view the use of medications as a short-term tool. I prefer to describe the use of medications as a possible adjunct to the therapeutic process. In my view, medication is accountable for only five percent of the results. When working with already labeled patients, it is important (as with any patient) to shift the focus from symptoms to the person's story. There you can find exceptions, past successes, and resources.

Psychiatric diagnosis is the only medical diagnosis without lab workup, biopsy, or other medical confirmation. Diagnosis is required to prescribe psychotropic medications; this is why diagnosis is crucial for drug companies to keep selling their products. If you view patients as people who need medications because of their neurobiological deficits, then medications are used as a long-term use. As Bill O'Hanlon says, when you give a label to something, you give this something a life on its own. The result of adding the term "chronic" to the label is an ongoing self-fulfilling prophecy. Under those conditions, medications are unavoidable long-term tools.

It's a question of viewpoint: The way you view patients determines the way you treat them. Being fond of the constructivist approach, I would like to mention a story that Betty Edwards, the author of *Drawing on the Right Side of the Brain* [1989] told me.

Betty developed a method for teaching drawing in which the early lessons consist of copying a drawing by laying it out upside down. It is much easier and more efficient to learn this way since we are unable to place the image in any known category (face, landscape, car, etc.). Our mind quietly and faithfully executes the contours of the subject it's reproducing. Ms. Edwards demonstrates in a brilliant fashion that by adopting this method, people who have convinced themselves that they can't draw, succeed at achieving results far beyond their expectations. The assertion of "I don't know how to draw" collapses.

Edwards understood that this "natural" tendency to put things into categories destroys individual creative powers. She became curious about the functioning of the brain and went to interview Roger Sperry, a neurologist who won the Nobel Prize in medicine for his work on "split brains." She learned that to be able to draw, it was necessary to quiet the left cerebral hemisphere and therefore activate the right hemisphere. She also observed the dominance of the left hemisphere. A strategy such as placing a drawing upside-down in order to copy it succeeds in silencing the left side. The problem is apparently trickier when it comes to drawing a person or a landscape directly because it is difficult to turn them upside-down. While we cannot put the world upside down, we can succeed in modifying our interpretation of "reality" by quieting the left brain and learning to use our creative resources. In therapy, we have to process the same way: Shut the analytical left brain and shift the attention to the whole person and the situation in which we meet the person.

One day, years ago, Betty received a letter from a psychiatrist who had been following her method to learn how to draw. He was a consultant in a hospital in the unit for patients diagnosed as depressed. He saw each of his patients at least once a week. Unfortunately, the patients remained fixed in the silence that is typical of people with depression. Discouraged and feeling that his therapeutic efforts were in vain, he did not have much hope left for curing his patients. Meanwhile, he was looking for models to use for his drawing training. He came to the point of filling his consultation time by asking his patients if they would let him do their portraits in exchange for a photocopy of the drawings. To his surprise, no one refused his offer, and his consultations were transformed into modeling sessions. From time to time he would ask them to turn their heads slightly, to move a strand of hair out of their eyes, or he would compliment a certain facial feature. The heavy silence of the old sessions was transformed into an atmosphere of artistic concentration. After three weeks, he was happily surprised to see that all his patients were doing much better. Smiles were no longer a rarity, men shaved and trimmed their beards and mustaches, and women put on makeup and became coquettish again. According to the psychiatrist, this unexpected therapeutic effect was due to his patients not experiencing themselves as patients anymore, but in their new role as models, they perceived themselves as being fully human. He finished his letter by thanking Betty Edwards for the quality of her lessons and for her indirect influence on his work. She wrote back to say that she was enchanted by the unexpected effect that he had obtained by drawing his patients, and that they most likely improved because they were no longer defined as patients but rather as models. She added that in her opinion, he had transformed the view of his role as psychiatrist and therefore changed his behavior and attitude toward his patients and this had certainly contributed to their success.

This is a demonstration of the impact that the construction one has of oneself can have on the construction of others in relation to themselves. To come back to the question of medications used as a short- or long-term tool, I like the concept, "tool." A tool doesn't make the craft of the therapeutic process; it might help only if correctly used and seen as what it is: a tool and not a one-size-for-all solution.

CONCLUSION

Joel often has joked that mental health practice might have been better off had Freud been a plumber. Instead, psychotherapy practice has fallen under the rubric of medical practice. As a result, clients are fitted to practice rather than practice fitted to clients. Medicine seeks physiological causes to symptoms. The patient seeks out the physician; the physician forms a range of possible explanations for the malady and then performs tests in order to identify the most probable cause. Based on the results, the physician prescribes a treatment or series of treatments. If the prescribed course alleviates or cures the symptoms, then the treatment has been successful. If not, the physician needs to reinvestigate either the diagnosis or the treatment—problem solving at its most effective.

Unfortunately, mental health is more ethereal. Efforts to concretize psychiatric symptoms have been less than a resounding success. As Thomas Szasz (1979) reminds us:

> It is important to keep in mind that, at the beginning of his career, Freud thought of himself as a psychopathologist. Accepting the literal reality of mental diseases, he sought to discover their causes or "etiologies . . ." (p. 125)

When he failed to do so, Freud devised a complex theory in an attempt to explain what he was observing in his consulting room. Szasz continued:

> Why was Freud so exuberant? Because he hit upon the formula that enabled him to be free, once and for all, of the burden of tailoring his theories to fit the facts of external reality. Henceforth, he could fit the facts to his conjectures. (p. 128)

Ever since, the number of theories addressing the causes and proper treatment of mental illness have steadily proliferated. According to Miller, Duncan, and Hubble (1997), about 500 different theories of psychotherapy exist. Even though each one professes to be the true and right path, in reality, outcome data suggest that no one theory is superior to any other. Beutler et al. (1986) stated,

> For example, the wide differences between process and outcome findings with respect both to therapist status and global theoretical orientations suggest that these two concepts have limited value for directing future research. In both of these cases, a wide variety of treatment outcomes have been explored with little indication of meaningful difference emerging. (p. 297)

Yet the consistent and almost obsessive focus on devising the right model that will somehow be the key to unlocking the mental illness treatment door has done little but create a muddle. Although, no doubt, the treatment of users of the mental illness system has become vastly more humane and arguably more effective in the past 100 years, the main, current practice serves to co-construct pathology and *dis*ability.

When we talk about diagnosis with clients, how much are we actually co-constructing a way of life rather than identifying some true medical condition? How much are we constructing clients as their labels rather than as humans who experience successes, talents, and skills in addition to distressing thoughts, feelings, or behaviors? The very word *symptom* suggests something deep and disturbing. In SFBP, we believe that all behaviors, thoughts, and feelings exist within contexts and are made meaningful in those contexts. Those same contexts contain a plethora of other thoughts, feelings, behaviors, people, relationships, and meanings that can be used to make sense of the complaints in a different light, often illuminating them in ways that make them disappear or that reveal possible solutions that may seem counterintuitive within a paradigm of pathology.

All four psychiatrists who were interviewed bring a refreshing message. Rather than listening to diagnoses, rather than listening to pathology, they have chosen to listen to their patients. Each of them in his or her own way has chosen to develop conversations that construct hope and possibilities, conversations that make patients' resources and strengths "real."

No one is born aspiring to spend their lives in treatment for mental illness. We are all born with the capacity to imagine and hope for a satisfying and productive life, imagination, and hope that often have been buried under the weight of diagnostic labels and concomitant treatments. All four psychiatrists work with clients in a way that constructs conversations that tap into the energy inherent within the patient's imagination and hope.

NOTES

1. The authors' favor a "both/and" rather than an "either/or" perspective. The client can co-construct that both medication *and* doing things on his or her own are helpful. Our interest is how we engage the client in a conversation that promotes solution-building.

Chapter 8

Meta-Systemic Considerations of the Solution-Focused Brief Approach: Using the Ideas to Implement Solution-Focused Practices in Agencies and Hospitals

JOEL'S EXPERIENCES

Joel has had relevant experiences developing programs utilizing SFBP. In the first, as a director of a community mental health clinic in a private, not-for-profit agency, he was successfully able to convert a program that had utilized a conventional approach to one that was more solution-focused. Joel supervised the clinic for approximately nine years, about seven of which were solution-focused.

The process that led to the conversion of the clinic is illustrative. At the end of March 1992, Joel had been in the midst of training with the New York Milton H. Erickson Society for Psychotherapy and Hypnosis. The county, searching for more efficient ways of managing caseloads and waiting lists in their clinics, had become interested in the solution-focused approach. County clinical staff were required to attend a five-day training. Several supervisors from private community mental health clinics also were invited. Joel was included in this group.

Excited by what he was learning, Joel was eager to test the approach in actual practice. He returned to his clinic, and the staff agreed to attend a three-day solution-focused training during which Joel would show them what he had learned. Joel suggested that if, after the training, the staff members were interested, they would continue, eventually working with clients using the new approach.

Solution-Focused Brief Practice
© 2007 by The Haworth Press, Taylor & Francis Group. All rights reserved.
doi:10.1300/5507_08   *133*

In fact, the staff were very interested and they continued to role-play, inviting Joel's supervisor to act as a client. At that time, the clinic did not have a one-way mirror. Using the agency's VCR and television monitor, Joel brought in his own video camera from home with a tripod. The VCR and monitor were placed in Joel's office with the camera in a colleague's adjacent space. A long patch cord was purchased and attached between the VCR and camera so that the observing team could view the session. The office was too small to include both the therapist and client in the view, so the camera was focused solely on the client.[1]

During the course of this trial period, staff from other programs who were also interested in the solution-focused approach attended sessions and participated with the consulting team. In the opinion of the authors, the use of team sessions and the influence of the external colleagues served to reinforce and maintain a solution-focused stance. Another major factor that reinforced solution-focused practice was the discussions of what staff members in general were defining as positive outcomes. In fact, most of the staff members involved in those early experiences still practice a solution-focused approach.

Eventually, the county decided to privatize one of their clinics. The agency Joel worked for applied for and was awarded the clinic, and Joel was asked to take over directorship of the newly acquired program. Fortunately, the former county clinic had a large room that was separated from a smaller therapy office by a one-way mirror. Joel hired staff that had either been exposed to solution-focused practices or were willing to be trained in and use the approach.

Six months after Joel's initial training, he was introduced to Dan Gallagher. Dan had been using the solution-focused approach for many years, including as the director of a state outpatient substance abuse clinic. He also had been a solution-focused trainer and consultant. Joel hired Dan as a consultant, and he met with staff monthly. Unofficially and on his own time, Dan often came to the clinic and participated behind the one-way mirror.

During the time that Joel supervised the program, the clinic garnered a reputation as a place where other professionals could observe behind a mirror and see the approach in action. Visitors came not only from the United States, but European countries as well. When Insoo Kim Berg visited the clinic in May 1998, she commented that the clinic was reminiscent of the Brief Family Therapy Center in the early 1990s.

While in the clinic, Joel began a series of three-day solution-focused trainings for agency staff, not only in the clinical division, but in the residential and employment divisions as well. These trainings were well attended, and feedback by attendees indicated that the trainings were useful to them in their positions. Several commented that the trainings challenged their long-held beliefs.

As the clinic continued to operate from an SFB perspective and Joel continued to periodically offer trainings, professionals outside of the agency began to call, asking to participate in the trainings. Toward the end of Joel's tenure with the agency, the participation percentage began to tip in favor of those outside of the agency's employment. This provided another source of income for the agency.

Because the clinic was one of four operated by a larger agency that also provided employment and residential services, and because the various clinics were networked on a central computer database, Joel was able to compare data from his clinic with other agency clinics that operated from a more traditional psychodynamic approach.

Comparative Data

Joel compared data from two clinics operated by the agency during the period of April 1997 through April 1998. Tables 8.1 and 8.2 show the comparisons between the two clinics. The clinics were similar in terms of the number of clients served. Clinic I used a traditional, psychodynamic orientation to therapy, and clients were expected to

TABLE 8.1. Comparative Analysis of Two Clinics' Intakes and Cases Opened. April 1997 to April 1998

	Intake	Number cases opened	Total cases	Intakes, average per FTE*	Cases opened, average per FTE	Total cases per FTE
Clinic I	363	418	781	145	67	77
Clinic II	816	857	1673	284	138	145

*FTE = full time employee

TABLE 8.2. Comparative Analysis of Two Clinics: Billable Sessions. April 1997 to April 1998

	Billable sessions	Billable sessions, therapists only	Average billable hours per FTE
Clinic I	5,796	3,408	631
Clinic II	5,968	4,500	763

attend weekly sessions. Clinic II was the one that Joel supervised, using a solution-focused approach.

The results demonstrate that the clinic that utilized a solution-focused approach served more than twice the number of clients as the more traditionally based unit and nearly twice as many clients per full-time employee. The results also indicate that the solution-focused clinic produced 132 more billable units than the traditional clinic during the one-year period. The clinic reimbursement came from three major categories: Medicaid, Medicare, and managed care. Self-pay clients produced a minor source of income with the majority paying the ten dollars base fee from a sliding scale. Taking into account all four income sources, we conservatively estimated average reimbursement to be approximately $45.00. This would suggest that the solution-focused clinic would have produced just a little less than $6,000 of income more than the more traditionally operated clinic during that one year.

Fairview Psychiatric Hospital

In early summer of 1999, Joel was interviewed by the director of a private, inpatient, psychiatric hospital. Although the director was not acquainted with solution-focused ideas, she expressed excitement at the possibilities as Joel outlined the approach. She asked him how he would go about converting an established adult unit to SFBP and Joel obligingly explained the process he would advocate. Joel reasoned that he would need to recruit from existing hospital staff, and he advocated a series of two-hour, in-house, solution-focused introductions. He suggested that at the end of each presentation, he would obtain a list of staff members who expressed interest in the approach and willingness to adapt it to the hospital.

Once staff members were recruited and chosen, they would engage in a three-day orientation to SFBP, during which they would have the opportunity to learn and practice the approach in depth. On-site supervision would reinforce the approach as staff members applied the approach to patients. Joel suggested that recruited staff, once trained and oriented to SFBP, would spend several days designing a solution-focused unit. The hospital utilization reviewer would be involved to ensure that the practice and, specifically, documentation, met licensing and accreditation requirements. Forms that were proposed would also be reviewed with the state office of mental health representative to further assure compliance. Joel estimated that the entire process would take between three and six months.

The administrator offered Joel a position with the understanding that he would establish a solution-focused adult unit. During the course of the next six months, Joel had the opportunity of observing and participating in a conventional inpatient psychiatric hospital in operation.

Joel reasoned that the administrator, his supervisor, needed to fully understand the solution-focused approach if the plan were to be successful. Although he had originally sent her several articles prior to his employment, she admitted she had never read them. She was urged and agreed to attend the training; unfortunately, her responsibilities precluded her doing so.

Joel began his tenure as treatment coordinator in August 1999. Per his blueprint, he organized a series of solution-focused trainings. These were completed with existing hospital staff as well as newly hired staff members. Joel attempted to organize a three-day training; however, because of the constraints of time and coverage issues, this was reduced to two days. Also because of coverage issues, staff members who had expressed interest were unable to attend. A social worker from the adult unit did attend for the morning of the first day but was called back to the unit in the afternoon and did not attend the second day's training. Another training was scheduled and no one attended, again because of coverage issues.

Joel convinced Dan Gallagher to join him in the endeavor, and Dan was hired part-time to help Joel develop the unit. In November 1999, Joel and Dan were asked to see the administrator. She announced that she had discharged the clinical staff in the adult unit and that Joel and Dan were to administer the therapy program beginning the next day.

Joel and Dan began to work in the adult unit with the established medical staff. Because of existing staff's training and orientation to the medical model, much of what Joel and Dan did was experienced by them as being outside of customary practice. None of the existing staff had attended either the solution-focused orientation or two-day training.

Several situations serve to illustrate the practical ways in which a solution-focused philosophical orientation differs from the medical model. Typically, when patients were first admitted to the unit, they spent the first day or two self-sequestered in their rooms. This especially was the practice when they were experiencing situations that they perceived as hopeless and without possibilities. The unit staff would urge them to join the unit activities, and when the patients demurred, they were characterized as noncompliant and resistant. The staff's training dictated that unless clients were engaged in activities led by hospital staff, other activities were irrelevant and even hindrances to their treatment.

On the other hand, Dan and Joel began with the assumption that whatever a patient does can be co-constructed with the therapist as useful and therefore sensible. When patients finally did emerge from their rooms, they would meet with Dan and Joel. They expressed interest about what the patients had thought about during the one or two days they spent in their rooms. Joel and Dan were amazed to learn that the majority of patients typically had made useful sense of their situations and had developed reasonable strategies for getting themselves back on track.

In another episode demonstrating the contrast between the medical model and solution-focused practice, a client who had been readmitted to the unit a number of times was sitting near a table located adjacent to the nurse's station. As she sat by herself, consistent with her usual behaviors while in the hospital, she was holding a lively conversation with no one visible. The daily progress notes[2] completed by the nurses contained statements such as, "Patient demonstrating schizophrenic behaviors" and, "Patient is responding to auditory hallucinations."

Driven by his curiosity, Joel asked the patient how it was helpful for her to talk to herself. She replied that it seemed to calm her down. The patient was then asked how she managed to calm herself down outside of the hospital and, at the same time, stay out of trouble. She replied, "Oh, I never do this outside of here; I just talk to myself in the hospital." From the patient's perspective, the activity of talking to herself was self-soothing and acceptable in the hospital context. From the hospital medical staff's point of view, the behavior was indicative of schizophrenia. The language games that we exist in at any given time result in effects that make sense within those games. Joel assumed that the patient's behavior made sense and in some way was useful to her. The medical model contains assumptions that clients enter the hospital with psychiatric illnesses and concomitant behaviors; therefore, behaviors are expected to be dysfunctional and symptoms of a psychotic process rather than useful in some way. Most people working within a medical model do not even think about how such behaviors might make sense within the client's context and are useful in some way.

This idea is reminiscent of the article "On Being Sane in Insane Places" by D.K. Rosenhan (1973). Rosenhan described the experiences of eight "sane people" who had gained admission to 12 different hospitals. The "pseudopatients" were instructed to tell the assessors that they were hearing voices.

> Asked what the voices said, [they] replied that they were often unclear, but as far as [they] could tell they said "empty," "hollow," and "thud." The voices were unfamiliar and were of the same sex as the pseudopatient. (p. 64)

All other data given to the evaluating staff were factual. All 12 pseudopatients were admitted to their respective psychiatric hospitals and labeled as schizophrenic. Initially, they kept secret diaries of their experiences for fear of raising suspicions. In time, they began to write notes openly; these behaviors were recorded in their charts, apparently more evidence of their "psychopathology."

Dan and Joel continued the practice of providing a therapy group each morning, using a solution-focused approach. Newly admitted clients were asked the miracle question, and established clients were asked scaling questions. Each session began with the question of what was already improving, and the orientation was toward discharge and a better life outside of the hospital milieu, not on symptoms and illness. Clients typically were asked to scale their readiness for discharge, who else in their families was noticing the improvements, and what would be different when they left the hospital so that they probably would never need to be hospitalized again.

One of the mental health aides, who came onto the unit in the evenings, expressed an interest in Dan's and Joel's approach and was open to leading a "scaling group" each evening. With minimal training from Dan and Joel, he met in a group with the unit's patients and asked them to scale their levels of improvement during the day. The patients stated that this was very helpful because the groups encouraged them to notice what was improving during each day.

Prior to Joel's and Dan's involvement in the unit, there was no separate space to meet with clients. Joel and Dan were able to commandeer an unused patient room in which to work. They worked as a team, one doing the interview while the other observed and provided input for compliments during the break. The observing partner remained in the room during the interview. The clients accepted this arrangement. On one cold December day, the heating system in another room failed, and the hospital removed the heating elements in the room used by Dan and Joel. They persisted, however, because it was the only private place to meet on the unit and everyone wore coats in order to keep warm.

Working from a solution-focused perspective inevitably results in brief treatment. de Shazer did not intend to develop a brief approach (personal communication, July, 1994). He had been interested in developing an approach based on empirical evidence gathered from direct work with clients.

This certainly was the case with the solution-focused work in the hospital. Hospital stays began to decrease and clients began to express their readiness for earlier discharge. This development resulted in palpable concerns on the part of the medically trained staff who, by nature of social construction, perceived that patients were expressing "flights into health." The hospital management expressed concerns because they deduced that shorter hospital stays would result in less income. One of the vice presidents of the parent institution came to Fairview Hospital for a management meeting and stated that patients should be encouraged to stay longer in order to "maximize their treatment."

Responding to institutional concerns, Joel and Dan arranged for a discharge committee composed of the hospital's head nurse and several of the medical staff on the unit whose purpose was to meet three times per week and help with discharge planning for patients who thought that they were ready for discharge. For the most part, this was a successful maneuver, taking the onus of briefer stays off Joel and Dan—at least temporarily.

Unbeknownst to Joel, when he was first employed, the hospital had experienced serious financial difficulties. Joel and Dan left the hospital in January 2000. On the day Joel and Dan left, the administrator expressed her regrets that due to financial difficulties, the hospital could no longer afford to continue employing them. The administrator continued that she had observed a major difference in the adult unit since Dan and Joel began providing services there. She explained that prior to their arrival, patients had complained that they were not being provided with therapy. More recently, patients had been complimenting the hospital on the quality of clinical services.

The hospital ceased operations not long after Dan's and Joel's departures. From the perspective of the hospital, Joel's attempt to establish a solution-focused program within the hospital was less than successful. Yet, for the purposes of this chapter, the lessons learned were valuable and, combined with what Joel had learned in his prior successes, may help to establish a blueprint for those daring (maybe foolhardy) enough to attempt similar projects.

In the preparation of this book, the authors interviewed individuals from two successful programs using a solution-focused approach. The first, Teri Pichot, supervises a drug treatment program in Colorado. The second, the University of Colorado Hospital (UCH), has successfully run a solution-focused inpatient adult psychiatric unit for more than 14 years. The next two sections of this chapter include information on how Pichot and UCH established their programs; how they mollify the financial people (for most accountants, solution-focused practice is counterintuitive); how they are able to work with professionals outside of their programs (especially judges, probation officers, and child protective personnel who mandate clients); and how they train, maintain, and recruit staff.

Jefferson County Department of Health and Environment

The Substance Abuse Counseling Program of the Jefferson County Department of Health and Environment in Lakewood, Colorado has been utilizing a solution-focused brief approach to the treatment of substance abuse since early 1995. Prior to its current program manager, Teri Pichot's, tenure, the program used an "eclectic approach" built around whatever approaches the therapists thought would be most effective. According to Pichot, the transition to a program based on the solution-focused brief approach took two or three years.

Teri Pichot was interviewed for this chapter in August 2004.

JS: Why was the shift to SFBT considered at the time?

TP: There was a question of how effective the program was in treating clients and even some discussion about terminating the program prior to the time I took over as program manager.

JS: What was the process like that led to the transformation to SFBT?

TP: I began asking the staff solution-focused questions and was careful not to act as the expert on doing therapy. We used video tapes of Insoo Kim Berg and Steve de Shazer, and engaged in role-plays. I would ask the staff questions about what was happening in therapy that was working from the client's point of view. Initially, the staff didn't have answers, but the questions caused them to be curious. The other question I would pose to them was, "What do you think would happen if you posed the same questions to your clients?"

When I became the program manager, we had six staff. About half of those remained through the transition period. The other half left, I think because they experienced the questions I was asking as critical of their practice. Those that remained did so because they were open to looking at themselves and became curious. That curiosity was contagious.

JS: How were staff recruited and trained?

TP: We didn't have much success advertising specifically for solution-focused therapists. Around here, everyone seems to think that they're solution-focused—confusing motivational interviewing [e.g., Cordova, Warren, & Gee, 2001] with solution-focused therapy. I found that the best way is to present solution-focused concepts to outside groups and notice who might be interested. What also happened was that the word got around after the presentations and prospective staff inquired about possible positions. Because interns are trained in SFBT while they are in our program, they also represent a good resource for prospective therapists.

JS: What modalities are used in your program?

TP: We use mainly groups, but also offer couples' and individuals' therapies. Clients decide on the length of treatment, with the exception of mandated clients who are court ordered. Mandated clients are also required to take urine screenings. Urine screenings are also offered and highly encouraged with all clients since they help them build trust with others and provide needed evidence that they are remaining abstinent; if they refuse, it's accepted.

JS: What were the reactions of clients to solution focus, especially those who were treated using more traditional approaches?

TP: In general, clients really like the approach. I think that's because we use their language. So, if they're twelve-steppers, we'll speak that language. I find that the twelve-step program can be integrated with SFBT.

JS: What about those who insist on going "deeper"?

TP: We ask if it's all right to begin by fixing the problem. I use the analogy, if you're lost in the woods, would you rather first figure out how to get out of the woods or sit, shiver, and figure out how you got lost. That helps them understand that taking action first would be most beneficial and that the insight will come after they take the necessary action.

JS: Do you work in teams and use a mirror?

TP: Yes, we find it especially useful to have a team behind the mirror during groups. We take a break and give feedback to the group members for the team. [Using] observing teams also helps maintain consistency of the approach.

JS: What seems to work to keep the program solution-focused?

TP: Primarily, a lot of supervision. I also meet with clinicians individually for an hour a week. The other element that works is using the mirror. We've found working this way keeps us energized. I use solution-focused questions in supervision, including the miracle question and scaling. For those staff members who are interested, there are a lot of opportunities to write about solution focus. Opportunities are given to interested staff to learn about administration and those who want to try training can.

JS: On a scale of zero to ten, how likely would the program stay solution-focused if you left?

TP: I would say, eight. My supervisor is sold on the approach. It wasn't always that way. She was skeptical until she saw it worked; now they offer the training to all staff within the health department. If I left, they would most likely recruit from within.

JS: How is the program funded?

TP: Some money from federal grants through the state. There are also some county funds, and we charge a fee on a sliding scale.

JS: In many ways, supporting a program financially while working briefly is counterintuitive. How did you convince the financial people that it would be a good idea to work this way? How do you convince them to keep working this way?

TP: I think the most important thing was that management saw that staff members were happier and they stayed. I don't fight regulatory requirements. I've learned to translate management's language into solution focus. I involved staff in solution-building around financial issues and paperwork issues. They decided to see more people and took turns covering for other staff who worked at home catching up on paperwork. They also decided temporarily to shift priorities to doing intakes.

JS: What about the outside systems—probation, DSS, the courts—how do they react to the program? How did you work with outside systems to make a solution-focused approach acceptable to them?

TP: My general rule is, don't answer questions unless questions are asked. We don't try to convert anyone and generally keep a low profile. I usually ask mandating agencies directly how they will know that the client is getting good help and how they will know that the client is finished with therapy. I don't use the term *solution focus*.

JS: What outcome data have you gathered?

TP: We've had high client satisfaction. When we've done surveys at discharge, clients comment that staff was caring and involved. Clients also complimented the kind of questions asked. The average stay was about six months. Of course, this number is skewed to the higher end because many of our clients are mandated to treatment.

JS: How many people do you see on a yearly basis? How does that compare to more conventional programs in the substance misuse field?

TP: We average about six hundred annually. I would estimate that other programs probably see more, but with higher staff dropout rates. We maintain a caseload cap of thirty-five clients per therapist.

University of Colorado Hospital

In 1994, the psychiatric unit of UCH began the process of converting to a solution-focused approach. The following interview was held by phone on August 9, 2004 with Bonnie Cox-Young, RN, MS, Senior Director for Psychiatric Services; Bari Platter, RN, MS, Clinical Nurse Specialist and Educator; and Judy Linn, RN, BSN, Nurse Manager for inpatient psychiatry.

JS: What was the unit before it went solution-focused?

UCH: In 1990, it was a traditional, locked, inpatient unit.

JS: Why the change to solution focus?

UCH: There were really two major factors. The first was the penetration of managed care into the Denver marketplace; that drove us to look into a different model. The second was feedback from our customers, who, for the most part, were self-insured, large corporations. We invited them to be part of discussions in designing this new program. We also looked at programs that were already being operated along similar lines like Massachusetts General. We were very much influenced by an article they had published in 1985. It was the changes in the marketplace and economics in the Denver area.

JS: What was it in Massachusetts and in your experience that got you to choose solution focus?

UCH: The model in Massachusetts was an intensive inpatient program. It was a model we called twenty-four hour care that was a step down from inpatient. It's now more familiarly called a partial hospital program. People would move quickly from intensive inpatient in a day or two or three, to a twenty-four hour care period. They would go to work during the day or in whatever they were involved with in the community. If they worked night shift, they would go to work at night.

JS: Why solution focus?

UCH: It's a good model. It focuses on the patient's strengths and stays in the patient's world. It made sense to us. It is a model that's not complicated and it puts patients in the center of care, identifying their needs. We could assist them to become independent again.

JS: What was the reaction of the staff in the unit prior to the change?

UCH: At best, it was mixed. Many staff members saw it as a loss. The biggest loss was you didn't get to see patients over a period of time and watch them doing better. As we moved people more quickly out of the hospital, the staff didn't get to see the improvement in the patients' conditions. I think another factor was just because it was a change. And in some ways, it was more work; you had less time and you had to provide more intense treatment to get goals accomplished. Another issue was the power differential really shifted when we implemented solution focus on the unit. Some staff who were raised professionally to expect a hierarchical relationship with patients had difficulty giving up the control of power. For those staff, it was hard for them to stay, and some left. For other staff, it was a relief to share responsibility for outcome and the work of treatment with patients being the center of that. We saw a split in the people who had difficulty giving up the control versus the people who really enjoyed a different kind of relationship with patients. The shift to solution focus really changed the structure of the programming and for the staff as well.

JS: What percentage of staff left because of the choice of approach?

UCH: We implemented it in two different places. We first implemented the approach on our managed/acute care unit—we call that the alternative program. There was no loss of staff. In fact, the staff was really excited about this new model. On the more traditional inpatient unit (mostly chronically mentally ill, public patients) there was some attrition because we had some longer-term staff who really were pretty invested in a power-based relationship with patients and couldn't adjust to the new approach.

JS: Any speculation why the difference in staff reaction between the two programs?

UCH: That unit was relatively new. It began in 1984 and the conversion to solution focus began in 1992. That was a factor. I think, also, the medical director of the alternative program was one of the driving forces behind it. So we had the cooperation of the medical staff. It was new and exciting for researchers in the university, so that was another factor for the acceptance. Also, we had hired a newer staff and we did extensive training with them. This was complemented by supporting paper work and the transition was very smooth with the staff very much involved. It was critical to make the transition to this model to have both hospital administration and medical staff buy in to the change. To me, this is the most critical point in having made this successful transition and something that has lasted over time.

JS: How did you convince management to go in this direction?

UCH: It was the beginning of managed care at that time. Traditional units were still having an extraordinary month-long length of stay. It was actually our medical director who promoted the idea that we could serve patients with a shorter length of stay. That was a major component for management to give us the approval. I was first in this position in 1989. We went to the new model in 1990. The medical director had been in the position for just a year. Neither of us was tied to an old model. There were some financial issues that began to arise, and this also was a hook that the medical director used to get hospital administration interested. We were able to convince them that we could get the business. In part, we built our referral base by talking to some of the corporations that were self-insured and soliciting their interests. So, I think we built those things and then sold it to hospital administration.

JS: In terms of recruiting staff, how did you do that?

UCH: Nothing out of the ordinary. We tried to make our ads solution-focused. We would use language like, "Come to an innovative, pioneering, state-of-the-art facility." We revised our interview tool to be solution-focused. In addition to providing solution-focused therapy to patients, we also adopted a solution-focused leadership style as well. We queried applicants on their strengths, their resources, what they brought to the setting, and their flexibility. Right from the beginning, everything was solution-focused.

JS: Did you specifically ask for people who knew solution focus or had training?

UCH: We knew there would be few people who had exposure to it. We did ask if they knew what it was, if they had any training, if they had worked in any environment where that model was used.

JS: How did you train the staff?

UCH: Initially, all the staff went through a sixteen-hour, solution-focused orientation. That included all the patient care staff: nursing staff, mental health workers, social workers, and other nonphysician clinicians. Now, because of financial constraints, all staff go through an eight-hour training day and they have periodic updates. The training includes history and implementation of SFBT in the hospital, overview of de Shazer's conceptual model as well as Scott Miller's [e.g., Duncan, Miller, & Sparks, 2000] work. I also include [di] Clementi's theory of change [cf. Miller & Rollnick, 2002] and have developed a tool that combines solution focus with change theory. For the first two or three years, we had someone from the Brief Family Therapy Center come out and do trainings. We did behind-the-mirror supervision. We had faculty from the University of Colorado Hospital School of Nursing attend as well as the leadership team.

We used closed-circuit TV. A staff member would interview a patient in front of the camera, we would watch on the TV and call to offer suggestions. There would be a therapeutic break where we would give the staff member a suggestion on an intervention. The staff person would go back in front of the camera to deliver the message. After the session we would use a parallel process. We would interview the staff member and identify their strengths and what they did well. We complimented them on what they were successful on and then offered some suggestions for improvement. That was a really great project that went on for a couple of years.

Commonalities

Based upon Joel's experiences as well as those of the Substance Abuse Counseling Program of Jefferson County Health Department and UCH, we can deduce key elements that increase the probability of a successful transition and operation of a program using a solution-focused practice.

Administrative Support

Those in the upper levels of management, especially those who are directly responsible for supervision of a program, need to know the meaning of solution-focused brief practice in detail. They need to understand and be prepared for the possible consequences that might come from conversion to a solution-focused practice. Both Jefferson County and UCH experienced attrition because a percentage of the staff could not accept the change. Administration needs to understand the loss as a very probable reaction and prepare for it. Management must set a priority for orientation and training of staff in SFBP.

Administration needs to be kept informed throughout the processes of design, implementation, and day-to-day program management. Administration needs to know that positive outcomes will make the difficult process of transition worthwhile. By soliciting the corporate clients of the solution-focused unit, the staff at UCH were able to demonstrate the advantages of converting the unit to SFBP to the administration in a very concrete way. Once the program is established, it is helpful for administration to have reinforcing information about positive client outcome data, meeting financial goals, and positive staff morale.

Consistency of Approach

Practice needs to be consistent. It makes little sense to maintain a problem-focused/medical-model language game and at the same time attempt to incorporate solution-focused principles. In order to successfully transition and maintain a solution-focused program, staff members need to accept and be trained in the approach. The system must have a consistency of approach throughout. Our own experiences suggest that attempting to mix solution-focused and problem-solving methodologies is a formula for confusion. Pichot, however, discussed the ways she accommodated medical model practices. It makes little sense to get into power struggles with administration and staff. Rather, taking time to demonstrate the approach at all levels of conversation seemed helpful to the Jefferson County program.

Several strategies have proven useful to successfully convert and maintain the solution-focused approach: preparation of administration and existing staff, quality initial training, feedback in the initial stages, periodic refreshers, ongoing solution-focused supervision, and, at least in the initial stages, the use of an observing team.

Quality Initial Training

Initial training has two major purposes. The first is to provide staff with the solution-focused tools that will allow them to begin practicing with clients immediately following the training. The second (and probably more important) is to orient staff to the solution-focused language game. During the course of this book, we have emphasized the differences between problem-solving and solution-building approaches, and these ideas should be used at all levels during the conversion.

Joel recalls that he once was introduced as doing a presentation on "solution-focused problem solving." It is usual for those being introduced to SFBP to attempt to understand it along the problem-solving continuum. Even those who have practiced it may find themselves reverting to problem solving. For example, when doing scales, we initially asked clients what they would need to do to move up one point on the scale. Understandably, the strategy was to make clients responsible for change. Alternatively, we began asking what would be different once they moved up one point on the scale, thus averting the whole question of agency of change—a problem-solving factor—and focusing more on the positive results of change.

Staff needs to realize the very palpable differences between problem-solving and solution-building. During three-day introductory trainings, it is very common to hear trainees express confusion at the end of the first day. Later, they reflect that it was around then that they began to realize the solution-focused approach is advocating something very different from what they were initially taught and often held sacred.

Thus, training needs to address both the practical and philosophical aspects of solution-focused practice. The balance is best achieved by a trainer who has had experiences and skills in teaching solution focus. If the organization has such a trainer, it may consider itself lucky. If not, it behooves the organization to seek out an established trainer.

Feedback in the Initial Stages

Our experience is that trainees typically leave trainings enthusiastic and eager to experiment with the approach. Clients, especially those about whom we wrote this book, have been well socialized in problem-solving thinking and conditioned to working with therapists from this perspective. When therapists initiate solution-building questions, clients respond (in accord with past experiences) in problem-solving ways. Novice solution-focused therapists often respond by reverting back to a comfortable problem focus. It is imperative that trainees be given the opportunity on a regular basis to review their practices and learn how to take the next steps. This can be accomplished only in the context of actual application of the approach to real clients and supervision with a knowledgeable and skilled solution-focused practitioner.

Periodic Refreshers

Just as quality initial training is important, so is having periodic trainings that highlight various solution-focused tools. For example, refreshers can be specific to the miracle question, scaling questions, formulating feedback to the client, or designing between-session tasks. Refreshers also can focus on application to specific clientele or, for example, substance misuse, clients who cut, symptoms such as hallucinations and delusions, and specific applications such as solution-focused group therapy. Presenters can be in-house therapists who have demonstrated a particular inclination or have had valuable experiences and successes to share with their colleagues. Presenters also can be outside "experts." Having agency staff members provide training reinforces the concept of doing more of what works and encourages staff by providing feedback that they are on the right track. Hiring outside presenters infuses staff with new ideas and refreshes a sense of excitement, new possibilities, and options.

Ongoing Solution-Focused Supervision

It is helpful for those who are newly learning to use solution-focused practices to be supervised on a regular basis by someone who is experienced in the approach. Supervision should utilize a solution-focused approach. The supervisor needs to be interested in what supervisees are learning that is helpful to clients and what supervisees perceive would be useful for them to learn. Solution-forced supervision (forcing trainees to use the solution-focused approach the same way as the supervisor) produces similar results to solution-forced therapy (Nylund & Corsiglia, 1994).

We often have found group supervision to be the most useful context for learning. Therapists learn from one another, thus taking the supervisor out of the expert role. In this context, the supervisor's task is to guide the process and set the parameters for learning. Early learners can attend the sessions on a weekly basis while more experienced therapists have the option of attending when they perceive that it will be useful for them. The purpose of supervision ultimately is to create a collegial support network.

The value of contact between therapists in the milieu cannot be overemphasized. It is our experience that informal conversations that colleagues have about successes and new learning serve to reinforce practice and enhance staff morale. Enlightened organizations find ways of structuring the workday and floor plan of the facility to enhance the probability of staff contact.

Use of an Observing Team

All three successful experiences detailed in this chapter described how the use of an observing team promoted and enhanced solution-focused practice, especially in the early stages of learning. The use of an observing team is valuable for both beginners and experienced practitioners on either side of the one-way mirror. As a therapist, knowing that the observing team is watching provides a sense of security as well as motivation to stay solution-focused. One is more likely to be circumspect about practice knowing that a group of colleagues is watching.

The usual conversation as part of the observing team is to note which questions are useful to the client. Team members typically discuss other questions they might have asked the client. Observing team members not only provide a resource for the therapist, but a parallel learning process takes place during the course of the session between what is going on in therapy and what is going on in learning and supervising.

If the agency is equipped with a one-way mirror with a quality sound system, so much the better. Earlier in this chapter, Joel explained in detail how his staff initially worked in teams using a video camera, VCR, and television monitor. With the client's written permission, sessions can be taped and reviewed later. As a way of using tapes, Insoo Kim Berg (personal communication, October, 1999) suggested that the staff member choose two ten-minute segments. The first would highlight an intervention that the therapist perceives was useful for the client. The therapist would choose a second segment that would pose a question for discussion.

As explained previously, without the availability of a second consultation room, Dan and Joel worked together with one acting as the observing team in the room where the session was being held. We have had clients who have requested that the team be in the room. Although this is not ideal, because the team does not have the ability to discuss the session without disturbing the client, it is an alternative if a second room is not available.

Staff Commitment

Involving staff in the design and implementation of a solution-focused practice offers several advantages. Staff members bring with them a variety of experiences and opinions that infuse a system with fresh ideas and perspectives. In addition, staff members who are actively involved in the designing and implementing process experience a greater commitment and willingness to make it work. Pichot described how she had times when her staff's flexibility and brainstorming made the crucial difference during those periods when the program was confronted by financial and administrative concerns. If the program is to work, staff needs to be committed to developing solutions. The most practical way of enhancing staff commitment is to involve them in all phases of implementation and operation of the unit.

It Is Solution-Focused, Not Solution-Forced

Solution-focused practice consists of assumptions, philosophy, and intervention tools that have been shown to be useful for engaging people in useful conversations. It is not useful to construe SFBP as the answer to all the woes that beset the world. As solution-focused practitioners, we do not perceive ourselves as obliged to convert all nonbelievers to the approach. The essence of the SFBP approach is a deep respect for the resources, abilities, and worldview of those with whom we work. This not only includes our clients, but also extends to our colleagues and the intra- and intersystems with which we communicate. It does little good to insist on shining the "light of truth" on those who hold a different view.

In our experience, Pichot's advice is well taken:

1. Keep a low profile.
2. If the community has negative attitudes toward the approach, it is probably best not to refer to what is being practiced as "solution-focused."
3. Listen and respond to the concerns of outside systems.
4. Invite staff to use a solution-focused approach to concerns raised by others.
5. Use others' knowledge and expertise about the client.
6. Find out from outside sources how they will know that what the program is doing is making a difference.
7. Compliment, compliment, compliment.

NOTES

1. At the 2004 Solution-Focused Brief Therapy Association conference, one agency presented a workshop in which they showed how they solved the viewing problem by installing a mirror behind the client so that the therapist and client could be seen simultaneously.

2. The more Dan and Joel worked in the hospital, the more they were curious that the term *progress notes* was used to denote something that did not seem to ever describe progress. In fact, when Dan and Joel actually noted progress. the hospital staff accused them of being in "la-la land."

Chapter 9

Philosophies that Inform Solution-Focused Brief Practice: Poststructuralism, Social Constructionism, and Language Games

> Where you stand determines what you see and what you do not see; it determines also the angle you see it from; a change in where you stand changes everything.
>
> de Shazer 1991, p. *xx*

The current viewpoint of the authors of this book on solution-focused brief practice and long-term users of mental health services can be described through philosophies of poststructuralism, constructivism, and social constructionism, as well as Wittgenstein's (e.g., 1958) ideas about language games. It is beyond the scope of this book to provide a comprehensive discussion of these and other ideas that inform the SFBP approach. However, because they are important to our understanding of the work described in earlier chapters of this book, we will attempt in this chapter to explain the fundamental ideas of the philosophies. Readers are referred to other works for more in-depth discussions related to philosophy of science and de Shazer's (1991, 1994) discussions of the ideas from which the approach sprung, which drive it, and which may describe it within a philosophical framework (esp. 1994).

Throughout this chapter, we will attempt to describe these ideas as they pertain to various aspects of the lives of people who have been diagnosed with a mental illness from a medical model perspective and have been in the psychiatric treatment system for a long time or

Solution-Focused Brief Practice
© 2007 by The Haworth Press, Taylor & Francis Group. All rights reserved.
doi:10.1300/5507_09

are expected to be in that system for some time into the future. Clients with certain diagnoses and the people around them often are told that their situations are "incurable illnesses" or "personality disorders," and they are led to believe that therapy needs to be interminable or that a lack of progress indicates that more therapy is needed—the fault of the client rather than the fault of the therapy or a fit between the two. In these cases, therapy becomes long-term because therapists, clients, and others in the clients' lives co-construct a reality of problems *or* solutions rather than situations of problems *and* solutions.

In the chapters of this book, we described situations in which so-called difficult problems disappear and no longer require therapy, in which complaints are no longer seen as problematic, and in which a client finds ways to reach goals and enjoy life even in the midst of ongoing distress. The first two situations suggest that therapy is no longer needed; the latter may suggest that therapy can continue, but not with a goal of "curing" the "illness" or of making the symptoms go away. Rather, the client's goal may be to continue to use mental health services as part of long-term management. The decision lies in what the client rather that the therapist thinks will be helpful.

PHILOSOPHY

de Shazer (1994) described two philosophies that inform solution-focused practice: poststructuralism and constructivism. He was careful not to attempt to develop a (capital T) Theory[1] of either how problems come about or how therapy works; philosophy gives light to description rather than explanation. In addition to continually observing and describing what clients were teaching him and Insoo Kim Berg, his wife and co-developer of the solution-focused approach, de Shazer was very interested in Wittgenstein's ideas about language and language games (the rules of conversation in which the context contributes to the meanings of words). He read extensively in philosophy, and his writings reflect this. However, his therapy focused on the pragmatics of listening to clients, learning from them how to be helpful, and writing about these practices. It is important to understand that the approach developed through de Shazer and Berg's and others' experiences of working with clients, not from philosophy. Philosophy is used to supply additional frameworks for the work.

This chapter will cover basic philosophical issues of poststructuralism, constructivism, social constructionism, and Wittgenstein's ideas of language games. Many books and articles cover the ideas more thoroughly, and we invite readers to avail themselves of these resources. These descriptions are our understandings of the ideas informed through the writings of others, including de Shazer, many conversations, and our own experiences. We make no claim that they are the only ways of understanding SFBP.

STRUCTURALISM

A structuralist philosophy is positivistic in that it is based on a view of the world wherein language represents reality (de Shazer, 1994); that is, a "true" correspondence exists between a word and what the word represents. For example, from a structuralist perspective, the word *chair* has some sort of direct relationship to that thing on which we sit. Of course, on one level, we know that this is true, that such things as "chairs" exist, and that if we ignore this fact, we deserve the pain we get when we stub our toes in the night. We also know, however, that the word is arbitrary, because other languages use different words or signs to mean the same thing. Nevertheless, the word itself has a certain "chairness." The structure of language requires this. We can understand what the word means by looking behind or beneath it for what it represents. Meaning thus is fixed by consensus among those using the language.

Similarly, from a structuralist perspective, such things as "borderline personality disorders" or "schizophrenia" exist that are related to the words that represent them. The words may be arbitrary, but they represent something real, and we can understand what the words are and what they mean by discovering specific aspects of clients' lives as they or others describe them. Hearing these descriptions from a structuralist perspective, practitioners use their theories to guide them in uncovering the underlying structures that support the descriptions, the "real" problems. These underlying structures then become the focus of therapy. Stephen's therapist, for example, might hear descriptions of David's difficulties in interactions with his mother and believe that David had underlying control or anger issues or that his "agoraphobia" rendered him helpless in certain situations. These issues, rather than the behaviors themselves, would be the focus of conversations. Another therapist might use the descriptions to diagnose poor self-differentiation (Bowen, 1978), and use this as the focus of therapy.

From a structuralist perspective, our jobs as therapists are, in part, to assess and discover "truth" by asking questions and eliciting descriptions of symptoms of underlying problems. The questions derive from the concepts of theories and elicit information that is consonant with those theories. Asking about childhood experiences, for example, is more likely to elicit evidence of lack of differentiation than would questions about current effects of the client's complaint.

When enough people use certain terms often enough, the words begin to mean not only what is observed, but they also suggest other things. For example, one of the main criteria for a diagnosis of a bipolar disorder is mania. Should someone be diagnosed with a bipolar disorder, she or he *must* be manic and, if not, simply does not know it . . . yet. Recall Joel's story about a man who lost his job and was subsequently diagnosed as depressed. His family history supported a diagnosis of depression, and his physician told him that he would struggle for the rest of his life. He took the prescribed medicine, became more lethargic, took to his bed, his wife informed his friends who stopped calling, and the man become more unable to function.

We often are amazed when people come to therapy because someone has diagnosed a difficulty that the client has not identified. One client came to therapy because she had told some co-workers that she had been molested as a child by her brothers. The co-workers had learned about childhood molestation and its consequences and were convinced that the woman needed therapy, despite that neither the client, her significant other, nor Thorana could determine anything whatsoever about her life that was so unsatisfactory as to require therapy. The client decided that the problem was her co-workers' worry, not the effects of the molestation. She rejected the idea that she was a "victim of abuse" because she did not feel abused. She explored the possibility that she *should* feel abused, but decided that although it was wrong of her brothers to treat her in such a way and that her relationship with them was different than it would be otherwise, she was functioning quite well. Using SFBP, we discussed what she could do to convince her co-workers that she was all right and would seek therapy in the future should she ever think she needed it.

From a structuralist perspective, so-called mental illnesses are medical problems that can be assessed and diagnosed by discovering them through the structures of symptoms and syndromes. Freud clearly was a structuralist when he described neuroses as a symptom of the failure of overwhelmed, inadequate, or fragile "egos" to mediate between "ids" and "superegos." Freud seemed to understand that these words were metaphors; however, many psychodynamic theorists and therapists have reified the terms to the point of nearly convincing themselves that ego, id, and superego are actual parts of brains.

Minuchin (1974), an early family therapist, understood the complaints that people brought to therapy as residing within family structures. Although he did not claim that these structures "caused" the problems, he was certain that the structures maintained the problems and that rearranging the family structures would make the problems go away. Minuchin looked less at the problems themselves and more at the underlying structure of the family, clearly defining him as a structuralist. His therapy (simplistically) consisted of changing the family structure so that the problem behavior would be resolved.

Similarly, the people at the Mental Research Institute (e.g., Watzlawick et al. 1974) saw difficulties as outcomes of interactions gone awry, of problematic communication sequences—another sort of structure. Their therapy consisted of helping people to interrupt the problematic interactions or to punctuate them in different ways that resulted in different perspectives in order to free the system from its homeostatic stuckness. This allowed it to move on in its natural development.

Modern-day medical views of mental illness look to the structures of the brain such as neural physiology and brain chemicals to explain the behaviors and thoughts of patients who act and think differently enough from the rest of society to cause concern, either for themselves or for others. Treatment providers with this view also tend to look to medicines to alter underlying physical and physiological structures. In all of these views of therapy, the required treatment is to alter the underlying structure, whether the structure is of the mind, family, relational interactions, or the brain.

We do not deny the validity of structural approaches to therapy. However, we believe that looking at people's problems this way is limiting and, worse, can lead clients and therapists to hallucinate or see structures for which they are looking as "really real," not as more or less useful metaphors. We believe that clients present us with many possibilities for describing difficulties and solutions.

POSTSTRUCTURALISM

Poststructuralism is based in postmodernism, and, different from structuralism, is a perspective that suggests that language is reality and that it cannot adequately represent what it purports to signify. In this view, no underlying structure must be understood in order to adequately communicate with others or ameliorate distressing behaviors. This is because what we perceive to be real is constructed through negotiating both problems and solutions. That is, we create rather than discover structures through language. It is clear that some things are real, regardless of what we call them—the chair, for example. If it hurts your toe when you kick it and it is used to sit upon, it must be a "chair."[2] Their purposes or usefulness, however, are not limited to "chairness" simply because we have now labeled the object. Staying with the object as "chair" may exclude other names—and therefore other purposes or uses such as "stool," "doorstop," or "playhouse."

Certainty our consensus of names applies to labels of mental illness. Indeed, the notions of "mental," "illness," and "mental illness" are no more real than "problems." Nothing is "real" about the *concept* of "chair"; its meaning is negotiated in social discourse, its context. What makes something a problem is not its structure, but the language or context in which it resides, including the description given to it by clients and others. The concept of "chairness" is outside both the word used and the way the word was constructed. Therefore, the way the word is can never completely capture its meaning; characteristics will always subtly defy description and meanings that are unique to specific situations. These characteristics become the focus of SFBP.

What is problematic for one person or system may or may not be problematic for a different person or system; furthermore, it likely is not problematic in the same way for everyone. For example, for some people, what is called bipolar disorder may be diagnosed and problematic because they dislike mood swings. For others, bipolar disorder may be problematic because it prevents them from doing the things they want to do. For yet others, it may be problematic because the people in their lives are distressed. Finally, for some, the behaviors that lead to a diagnosis of bipolar disorder are not problematic at all and may not be problematic until or unless someone labels them. Many artists (e.g., Schumann) may have done their best work during manic phases of what could easily have been diagnosed as bipolar disorders.

The conversations that people have about behaviors (as symptoms) and diagnoses make particular meanings about those behaviors and diagnoses. The day that my grandchildren use a chair to make a playhouse is the day that the word *chair* takes on a different meaning for them and for me. As Wittgenstein (1958) said, "For a large class of cases—though not all—in which we employ the word meaning, it can be defined thus: the meaning of a word is its use in the language" (p. 20). That is, the word *schizophrenia* has little meaning on its own—it is only a series of letters and sounds. In the context of language revolving around mental illness, however, it has particular meaning. In another context, such as a conversation about word derivatives, it has a very different meaning. Therefore, no particular or definitive meanings support the word *schizophrenia*. From a post-structuralist perspective, its meaning makes sense only in the context in which it is used. SFB practitioners, therefore, need to understand their clients' contexts as much as possible in order to understand clients' particular meanings about situations that they describe as problematic.

Similarly, differences in what is problematic are specific to people and their contexts; something is not problematic simply because it exists or because mental health professionals have identified it as a problem. The client was not a victim simply because she was fondled or had sexual intercourse with her brothers—that is a modern day construction of the situation. Similarly, no agreement exists about what causes schizophrenia, even though identifiable differences in brain physiology may exist in patients who have been identified as schizophrenic, and neither does agreement exist about what is the best treatment. Therefore, no specific structure underlies either the causes or the treatments of any of these situations. This illuminates a basic SFBP tenet: because no particular structure to problems must be discovered or unearthed, neither does a particular structure to solutions. In SFBP, the solutions identified by clients have more authority than anyone else's. Solutions are only solutions when they are employed by the client in the client's own life context and make a difference for the client.

An example of this idea from Thorana's therapy practice serves to understand the usefulness of a poststructuralist philosophy for therapeutic work. A client reported that she was anxious and that her anxiety was related to work stress. When asked what would be different when the stress and anxiety were no longer problematic for her, the client reported that she would feel more effective in her communication with her daughter, which had been frustrating for some time. We explored improving communication with the daughter and, after a few weeks, the client reported that work still was challenging, but that it was not causing her anxiety because it was not interfering with her relationship with her daughter. The hypothesized structure of the presented problem (anxiety due to work stress) did not provide necessary clues for solutions.

The client could have identified other aspects of her life that would be different and important, such as her enjoyment of her leisure time or her ability to sleep well. We could then have worked toward one of those as goals and found similar results. Therefore, the notion of the need to discover underlying structures of problems or of therapy is not necessary and is, in fact, limiting. It is possible to be effective by examining the issues that clients report rather than speculating on true causes or dynamics. Because we can work with the stated issue, the problematic dynamics supporting the problem do not need to be looked at, and focus can be placed instead on the goals that the client identified and a wide range of possible solutions can be explored. The therapist did not need to provide a definitive diagnosis, theory-derived goals, or specific solutions.

CONSTRUCTIVISM/SOCIAL CONSTRUCTIONISM

Maturana and Varela (1980), and von Glasersfeld (1987) espoused a philosophy of *constructivism*. In this way of thinking, reality is constructed by individuals through a process of making meaning of what is represented to the brain through the senses. According to these philosophers, no direct relationship exists between a thing and the meanings associated with it; therefore, there is no reality—only constructions. Radical constructivism, in our opinion, is of limited use in SFBP. We may believe that no such things as mental illnesses, chronic conditions, or long-suffering people exist, let alone real symptoms. Such an idea begs the question of whether or not schizophrenics would be mentally ill by themselves on deserted islands. The fact is, we are not on deserted islands, and symptoms, behaviors, thoughts, feelings, relationships, and chairs exist within contexts that are defined and described through interactions among people, ideas, beliefs, cultures, values, and history.

Social constructionism, as discussed by Gergen (e.g., 1985),[3] also suggests that meaning is constructed rather than inherent. For example, at some point in history, no concepts of "marriage" or "schizophrenia" existed. These concepts are constructed from data, similar to constructivism, but this process occurs in social discourse (language) and interactions (another kind of language) with other people, not simply between a phenomenon and a brain. We interact with others and therefore we construct, integrate, and synthesize meanings of phenomena within our social lives. Meanings may be consensually derived, but also are fluid and changing even as we speak about them. The act of speaking itself changes them. In interactions with others, we have only language as the tool for making meaning. "The limits of my language are the limits of my mind" (Wittgenstein, 1922, p. 21). From this notion of constructed knowledge and meaning, it is easy to see that the meanings we give to problems and solutions are not inherent in the phenomena or even in the conversations we have about them. de Shazer looked to the language games described by Wittgenstein to help him understand how the conversations that people have shape definitions and descriptions of symptoms, solutions, and therapy. These conversations are between the therapist and the client, and neither alone can claim them. They are *co-constructed* between the client and the practitioner through the discourse of therapy, and are not immutable, even after therapy is over. The meanings derived in the therapy room continue to flow as the client and the practitioner move into interactions with others in their lives. Thus, as David responded differently to his mother as a result of his conversation with Joel, she responded differently to him, an interaction that further affected the meanings that David and she and Joel made about the interaction (an exception), their relationship (more like adults), and therapy (useful for helping to construct new frames that are helpful for David).

Similarly, the events, thoughts, behaviors, emotions, and relationships that people call problems are fluid and constantly changing. The advantage of this perspective is that in therapy, neither the therapist nor the client is above the other—each participates in the co-construction of both the problem story and the solution story. Neither is the ultimate expert on either the problem or the solution; each has equal responsibility and privilege in the therapeutic process. Therapy is not something that therapists merely do to clients. Rather, therapy is a particular kind of conversation and interaction between clients and therapists as they strive to understand and make meaning through each other's language and the therapy context.

Many question this idea. After all, are therapists not supposed to be highly educated and trained professionals who *know* about mental illness and treatment? We believe that rather than being experts in terms of theory (or Theory), problems, therapy, or clients' lives, we are experts in the conversation of a particular kind called therapy, responsible for our part of the process of helping clients construct or rediscover solutions to their difficulties. Clients, however, are the experts when it comes to their life contexts, their experiences, their goals, and workable solutions for their situations. They know their lives better than we do. They are the only ones who can describe their problematic situations and what would constitute better lives, and just because they utter the word "agoraphobia," we cannot know what this means to them. Of course, therapists in other kinds of approaches are experts on the kinds of conversations that they co-construct with their clients. Most of these are problem-focused or some sort of structure-focused conversations. SFB practitioners are experts on solution-building conversations and watch for openings related to solutions rather than problems or underlying structures. Thus, together, the client and the therapist co-construct a view of reality that focuses on solutions rather than on problems or structures.

The process of therapy is one of describing how clients experience their problems and of exploring exceptions to the problem as well as their goals for therapy. Through this process, we participate with clients in developing solutions that may not be like those for anyone else with similarly described problems, because they evolve from clients' experiences of exceptions, goals, and successes, not therapists'. In this matter, SFBP is unique. Neither do we have a theory of how these problems developed—to develop such a theory would not be useful because it would not necessarily tell us anything about solutions. We have no theory of how therapy works, because to have one would privilege our construction of therapy above the clients' and would reduce our usefulness to them. Rather, we focus on clarifying our understandings (or *mis*understandings, as de Shazer [1991] put it) of clients' problems, goals, and solutions as descriptions rather than as explanations. By asking questions and noticing certain things, we engage in a particular language game (Wittgenstein, 1958) with our clients.

In fact, it is not necessary for clients to define a problem in order to engage in a solution-focused conversation. Therapists do not need to know problems in order to engage in conversations with clients about how life can be more satisfying and rewarding. SFBP thus can be applied in a wide rage of human endeavors, including therapy, business, hospice practice, and supervisory relationships, to mention a few.

LANGUAGE GAMES

All of social interaction involves language games. Language games are the rules and grammar of different kinds of conversations and are the only tools we have for knowing about others' realities. Particular language games are related to law, accounting, music, and all other contexts for discourse. In mental health, many language games follow the rules of medicine. de Shazer (1994) described language as behaviors that include gestures, facial expressions, utterances, and silence, not merely words. Contexts and cultures have different rules for how language is used and how it is interpreted. The meaning of words is dependent on the contexts in which they are used and the rules for using them. Readers interested in the intricacies of this idea are encouraged to read Wittgenstein for themselves. For the present work, however, it is helpful to understand that (simplistically) language games describe problems, different ones describe solutions, and yet different ones describe particular ways of doing therapy. That is, psychodynamic or strategic therapists use different rules for interaction from SFBP therapists.

In SFBP, the language game is one of *solution-building* (De Jong & Berg, 2002). Therapists use words, gestures, utterances, silence, tone, and facial expressions to encourage talk that focuses on solutions more than problems. It is not the case that problems are ignored; rather, it is important to listen to clients so that (1) they do what feels important and good to them and what they believe they are expected to do, and (2) we can listen with our "solution ears" for opportunities to use solution-talk. Solution-talk or solution-building utilizes language rules that focus on exceptions to predictable phenomena given the problem, to what is working, to goals, and to descriptions of present and future lives without the problem. Problem-talk, according to de Shazer and colleagues (see References), although necessary for some clients, is less useful for resolving problems than is solution-talk. The assumptions, concepts, and practices described in this book are all used to foster solution-building and to help clients move toward their goals.

NOTES

1. de Shazer was particularly fond of discounting Theory as helpful in therapy. That is, he believed that ideas about how particular symptoms, behaviors, or interactional dynamics develop were not only unhelpful, but had the propensity to limit possibilities. However, he agreed that humans are prone to want explanations and are not satisfied with simple description. He called this way of thinking (little t) theory to signify that many theories about something could exist, but that one grand Theory is a fallacy of thinking and not useful.

2. The idea that the object can be used for purposes other than sitting appears in the book as we explored with clients how resources can be limited by the ways we talk about them and can be similarly enhanced by conversation. This seems to suggest that chairs can be used for purposes other than sitting.

3. We make no claims here that Gergen somehow invented the notion of social constructionism, although it is a prevalent idea in fields related to psychology. Gergen's ideas evolved through his studies of philosophy. Franklin's (1995) work is helpful regarding applications of constructivism and social constructionism in therapy.

Epilogue

Several years after his last contact with David, Joel happened to be shopping in a local supermarket. While there, he met David. David informed Joel that his mother had died and that he had returned to the home that he had inherited. David explained that he was receiving Social Security disability because of his psychiatric condition. David also informed Joel that in order to maintain his disability benefits he felt obligated to remain in therapy and was now seeing a therapist weekly. He announced, "I learned what my *real* diagnosis is. According to my therapist, I'm a schizophrenic." David never completed his computer education and returned to living a solitary life in which his diagnosis once more had become central to his life and identity. We are distressed by a system that seems to force people to retain their labels in order to survive. We believe that supportive work helps people function as best they can, and that the parameters of that work should be determined by the people doing the work in collaboration with clients, and should not be dictated by other systems. Ideally, those systems would support our work.

Joel once worked in an adolescent intensive day treatment program with a psychiatrist who was a self-avowed "bipolar disorder maven." Joel estimates that the psychiatrist labeled at least 75 percent of his teenage clients with bipolar disorder. The psychiatrist insisted that the adolescents needed to know the implications of their disease so that they could learn better how to manage their illness—a lifelong proposition.

In one particularly telling conversation, the psychiatrist commented that he could not understand how Joel could help the adolescents without knowing how they were being intrapsychically motivated. Joel's response was to remind the psychiatrist that research data indicate all theories are about equal in outcome. The psychiatrist emphatically insisted that his was not a theory. Joel asked him whether he had the ability to see into the minds of people and therefore the ability to know with certainty what they are thinking. It is a particular delu-

Solution-Focused Brief Practice
© 2007 by The Haworth Press, Taylor & Francis Group. All rights reserved.
doi:10.1300/5507_10

sion that seems to infect the mental illness field, whereby observations are mistaken for inferences. We often question whether diagnosis is reflective of behavior or whether behavior is reflective of diagnosis. It was somehow sad when teenagers state, "I'm a bipolar," and their conversations with others in the program are centered on comparisons of their respective psychiatric hospitalizations.

How we, together with clients, use language determines the meanings that we and clients ascribe to the events that happen in our lives and ultimately to ourselves.

> Today, people come to me bearing their diagnosis: *I am a child of a dysfunctional family. I am an alcoholic. I am a love addict.* These names are worn like shields, psychological coats of arms. They do not move, these names. They are cold and solid, like an epitaph. I am certain these names reveal little of our true nature. Beneath the stories, beneath the diagnoses, these are all children of spirit, beings fully equipped with inner voices of strength and wisdom, intimations of grace and light. But their clinical diagnoses prevent them from believing in their own wisdom. Such names suffocate people's unfolding and limit the breath of their spiritual evolution. (Muller, 1996, p. 16)

References

American Psychiatric Association. (1994). *Diagnostic and statistical manual of mental disorders* (4th ed.). Washington, DC: Author.

Anderson, H., & Goolishian, H. (1992). The client is the expert: A not-knowing approach to therapy. In S. McNamee & K. J. Gergen (Eds.), *Therapy as social construction* (pp. 25-39). London: Sage.

Barnhart, C. L. (Editor in chief). (1961). *The American college dictionary.* New York: Random House.

Bateson, G. (1972). *Steps to an ecology of mind.* New York: Ballantine Books.

Bavelas, J. B., McGee, D., Phillips, B., & Routledge, R. (2000). Microanalysis of communication in psychotherapy. *Human Systems, 11,* 47-66.

Berg, I. K. (2000). *Building solutions in child protective services.* New York: Norton.

Berg, I. K., & de Shazer, S. (1993). Making numbers talk: Language in therapy. In S. Friedman (Ed.), *The new language of change: Constructive collaboration in psychotherapy* (pp. 5-24). New York: Guilford Press.

Berg, I. K., and Dolan, Y. (2001). *Tales of solutions.* New York: Norton.

Berg, I. K., & Miller, S. (1992). *Working with the problem drinker: A solution-focused approach.* New York: Norton.

Berg, I. K., & Steiner, T. (2003). *Children's solution work.* New York: W.W. Norton.

Beutler, L., Crago, M., & Arizmendi, T. (1986). Research on therapist variables in psychotherapy. In S. Garfield & A. Bergin (Eds.), *Handbook of psychotherapy and behavior change* (3rd ed., pp. 257-310). New York: Wiley.

Booker, J., & Blymyer, D. (1994). Solution-oriented brief residential treatment with "chronic mental patients." *Journal of Systemic Therapies, 13*(4), 53-69.

Bowen, M. (1978). *Family therapy in clinical practice.* New York: Jason Aaronson.

Bushman, B. (2002). Does venting anger feed or extinguish the flame? Catharsis, rumination, distraction, anger and aggressive responding. *Personality and Social Psychology Bulletin, 28*(6), 724-731.

Campbell, J., Elder, J., Gallagher, D., Simon, J. & Taylor, A. (1999). Crafting the "tap on the shoulder": A compliment template for solution-focused therapy. *The American Journal of Family Therapy, 27*(1), 35-47.

Solution-Focused Brief Practice
© 2007 by The Haworth Press, Taylor & Francis Group. All rights reserved.
doi:10.1300/5507_11

Cordova, J. V., Warren, L. Z., & Gee, C. B. (2001). Motivational interviewing as an intervention for at-risk couples. *Journal of Marital and Family Therapy, 27*(3), 315-326.

Crawford, W. (2003). *How to get kids to do what you want: The power and promise of solution-focused parenting.* Florida: Humanics Trade.

Deegan, P. (1993). *Recovering our sense of value after being labeled mentally ill.* Presentation at the Mental Health Care Reform: An Opportunity to Redefine Our Roles and Relationships, October 18, 1993, Tarrytown, NY.

De Jong, P., & Berg, I.K. (2002). *Interviewing for solutions.* Pacific Grove, CA: Brooks/Cole.

de Shazer, S. (1985). *Coming through the ceiling: A solution-focused approach to a difficult case* [Video]. Brief Family Therapy Center. Milwaukee, WI: Brief Family Therapy Center. (120 minutes.)

de Shazer, S. (1984). The death of resistance. *Family Process, 23*(1), 11-17.

de Shazer, S. (1985). *Keys to solutions in brief therapy.* New York: Norton.

de Shazer, S. (1988). *Clues: Investigating solutions in brief therapy.* New York: Norton.

de Shazer. S. (1991). *Putting difference to work.* New York: Norton.

de Shazer, S. (1994). *Words were originally magic.* New York: Norton.

de Shazer, S. (1998). How come solution-focused brief therapists think diagnosis is so bad? Retrieved January 15, 1998, from http://www.brief-therapy.org.

de Shazer, S., Berg, I., Lipchik, E., Nunnally, E., Molnar, A., Gingerich, W., & Weiner-Davis, M. (1986). Brief therapy: Focused solution development. *Family Process, 25*(2), 207-222.

Dolan, Y. (1991). *Resolving sexual abuse: Solution-focused therapy and Ericksonian hypnosis for adult survivors.* New York: W.W. Norton.

Duncan, B. L., Miller, S. D., & Sparks, J. A. (2000). *The heroic client: A revolutionary way to improve effectiveness through client-directed, outcome-informed therapy.* San Francisco: Jossey-Bass.

Edwards, B. (1989). *Drawing on the right side of the brain.* New York: Tarcher.

Franklin, C. (1995). Expanding the vision of the social constructionist debates: Creating relevance for practitioners. *Journal of Contemporary Human Services, 76,* 395-407.

Gergen, K. J. (1985). The social constructionist movement in American psychology. *American Psychologist, 40,* 266-275

Hoffman, L. (1990). Constructing realities: An art of lenses. *Family Process, 29,* 1-12.

Holmes, S., & Cantwell, P. (1994). Social construction: A paradigm shift for systemic therapy and training. *The Australian and New Zealand Journal of Family Therapy, 15*(1), 17-26.

Korman, H., (1997). On the ethics of constructing realities. *Contemporary Family Therapy, 19*(1), 105-115.

Korman, H., (2004). The common project. Retrieved June 15, 2004, from http://www.sikt.nu.

Lambert, M. J. (1992). Implications of outcome research for psychotherapy integration. In J.C. Norcross & M.R. Goldfried (Eds.), *Handbook of psychotherapy integration.* New York: Basic.

Lee, M.Y., Sebold, J., & Uken, A. (2003). *Accountability for solutions: Domestic violence solution-focused treatment with offenders.* New York: Oxford University Press.

Maturana, H. R., & Varela, F. J. (1980). *Autopoiesis and cognition: The realization of living.* Boston: D Reidel.

McFarland, B. (1995). *Brief therapy and eating disorders : A practical guide to solution-focused work with clients.* Hoboken, NJ: Jossey-Bass.

Metcalf, Linda (1995). *Counseling toward solutions: A practical solution-focused program for working with students, teachers and parents.* West Nyack, NY: Center for Applied Research in Education.

Miller, G. (1997). *Becoming miracle workers: Language and meaning in brief therapy.* Hawthorne, NY: Aldine de Gruyter.

Miller, G., & de Shazer, S. (1998). *Wittgenstein for therapists* [Audio]. Milwaukee, WI: Brief Family Therapy Center.

Miller, G., & de Shazer, S. (2000). Emotions in solution-focused therapy: A reexamination. *Family Process, 39*(1), 5-23.

Miller, S., Duncan, B., Hubble, M. (1997). *Escape from Babel: Toward a unifying language for psychotherapy practice.* New York: Norton.

Miller, W. R., & Rollnick, S. (2002). *Motivational interviewing: Preparing people for change.* New York: Guilford.

Minuchin, S. (1974). *Families and family therapy.* Cambridge, MA: Harvard University Press.

Muller, W. (1996). *How then shall we live?: Four simple questions that reveal the beauty and meaning of our lives.* New York: Bantam Books.

Nylund, D., & Corsiglia, V. (1994). Becoming solution-<focused>forced in brief therapy: Remembering something important. *Journal of Systemic Therapies, 13,* 5-12.

Rosen, S. (1991). *My voice will go with you: The teaching tales of Milton H. Erickson, M.D.* New York: Norton.

Rosenhan, D. (1973). On being sane in insane places. *Science, 179,* 250-258.

Shotter, J. (1994). Making sense of the boundaries: On moving between philosophy and psychotherapy. In A. P. Griffiths (Ed.), *Philosophy, psychiatry and psychology* (pp. 55-72). Cambridge, England: Cambridge University Press.

Simon, J., & Berg, I. K. (1997). Solution-focused brief therapy with long-term problems. *Directions in Rehabilitation Counseling* (Vol. 10; pp. 117-127). Long Island City, NY: Hatherleigh.

Simon, J. K., & Berg, I. K. (2004). Solution-focus brief therapy with adolescents. In F. Kaslow (Series Ed.) & R. F. Massey (Vol. Ed.), *Comprehensive handbook of psychotherapy: Vol. 3. Interpersonal/Humanistic/Experiential* (pp. 133-152). New York: Wiley & Sons.

Szasz, T. S. (1970). *The manufacture of madness: A comparative study of the Inquisition and the mental health movement.* New York: Harper & Row.

Szasz, T. (1979). The lying truths of psychiatry. *Journal of Libertarian Studies, 3*(2), 121-139.

von Glasersfeld, E. (1987). *The construction of knowledge.* Salinas, CA: Intersystems Publications.

Watzlawick, P., Weakland, J., & Fisch, R. (1974). *Change: Principles of problem formation and problem resolution.* New York: Norton.

Weiner-Davis, M., de Shazer, S., & Gingerich, W. J. (1987). Using pretreatment change to construct a therapeutic solution: An exploratory study. *Journal of Marital and Family Therapy, 13,* 359-363.

Wittgenstein, L. (1922). *Tractatus logico-philosophicus.* Cambridge, UK: Cambridge University Press.

Wittgenstein, L. (1958). *Philosophical investigations* (3rd ed.). New York: MacMillan.

Index

Page numbers followed by the letter "f" indicate figures; those followed by the letter "t" indicate tables; and those followed by the letter "n" indicate notes.

Printed in the United States
by Baker & Taylor Publisher Services

Printed in the United States
by Baker & Taylor Publisher Services